"Having an aged
stances. But hav
an even greater 1
Antonio knows fir
til I actually lived with her that I was able to evaluate what I could offer' . . . 'It's our responsibility as children to help our parents.' "
—*Progress with Purpose*, 2002 Annual Report
Texas Department of Human Services

"*Mi Mamacita Tiene Alzheimer's* is such a vitally important book in addressing the unique needs of the Hispanic patient with Alzheimer's disease and the family caregiver dealing with the ongoing stressors. The book is a poignant portrayal of an illness that robs a person of one's being and results in stress in another person. Theresa Vasquez transmits her memoir of her mother and her own personal experiences to give us insight into a Hispanic family as they cope with a very difficult disease. For the past thirteen years we have provided a Stress-Busting Program for Caregivers for the community. We have come to realize that Hispanics deal with the challenges of Alzheimer's disease in different ways than many non-Hispanic families. The book will begin to address many of these differences in a very personal, meaningful and compassionate way."
—Sharon Lewis, RN, PhD, FAAN
Professor, Schools of Nursing and Medicine,
University of Texas Health Science Center—
San Antonio, Texas Clinical Nurse Scientist,
Geriatric Research, Education, and Clinical Center,
South Texas Veterans Health Care System

"Terry guides us with tenderness and some very good comic relief that makes this time seem almost enjoyable. Although much frustration and anxiety are part of the difficult issues, Terry walks us through with confidence and love for her mother. More information is always good and the manner in which Terry doles it out makes you feel comfortable with the 'A' sickness. We have a long road ahead with the care of our family members who will be

stricken with Alzheimer and this book is a very good step in the right direction."
—Belinda Arredondo
Board Member SALF
Board Member of Wolfe Trail Kids Kamp
Secondary Educator
Assistant Sales Consultant for National Publishing Co.

"*Mi Mamacita Tiene Alzheimer's* is a must-read book for all Latinos who are faced with taking care of a parent with Alzheimer's. The book is very interesting, captivating, and spiritual, presented in a culturally sensitive manner. It will make a great gift to lift someone's spirit during this very difficult time."
—Dr. Gloria G. Rodriquez
Founder, AVANCE Family Support
and Education Program
Author, *Raising Nuestros Niños*

"Hispanics are the fastest-growing segment of the U.S. population. This book will assist caregivers and their families to take care of persons with Alzheimer's. It is a 'must have' for every family that lives with the illness."
—Rudy Valenzuela, FSP, MSN, RN, FNP-C
President, National Association of Hispanic Nurses

"This touching, heartfelt, personal account vividly portrays the pain felt by a daughter who becomes her mother's primary caregiver when it becomes evident she has Alzheimer's disease. The anguish felt by Vasquez is palpable, yet she cushions her pain with humor. This book deals with issues faced by a growing number of baby boomers, with a special focus on the traditions of a Hispanic-American family. The colorful narrative is laced with Spanish words and sayings. I recommend this book to anyone who is faced with caring for a family member with Alzheimer's disease."
—Maria Ramírez de Arellano
Chief Operating Officer, Hispanic Heritage Foundation

"Part personal memoir, part 'how-to' manual, this story of a Mexican-American nurse's love and commuter-care for her *mamacita* will touch the heart of anyone who has struggled to take responsibility for an aged parent, especially one who lives far away."

—Carolyn M. Parr
Outreach Minister, Festival Church

"Mary Theresa Vasquez raises a critical issue of our time—namely the caring for our aging parents—in a most personal way. Having served one year residency for a chaplaincy in a convalescent home and being pastor for fourteen years, I am well aware of the needs of our aging parents. Whether from Alzheimer's or other conditions, this is a need that cannot be understated in our country. Her comment, "Respect your elders and youth will respect you," reflects the inherent need for us to care for one another regardless of our condition—something contrary to our throwaway culture. Thank you, Mary Theresa, for your efforts in this cause!"

—Jeff Wuertz
Pastor, Chesapeake Community of Hope

"The story provides a 'cultural and language perspective to caring for Hispanic elders that is rarely seen in the literature.' As CEO for Centro de Salud Familiar La Fe, a large multi-health and -human services organization serving over 40,000 Hispanics, we applaud the contribution this book will make to holistic and culturally supportive care of Hispanic elders. 'La Fe' (faith), culture, love of family, and support in coordinating a maze of multiple health services is threaded together in a compassionate story of caring and resiliency."

—Salvador Balcorta, M.S.S.W., L.M.S.W.
Chief Executive Officer, Centro de Salud Familiar La Fe

"This is a must-read for anyone who is facing the challenges of caring for their parents as the aging process slowly expresses its true nature. . . . In the long run, we each are faced with a decision. And as this book clearly points out, either race, color, creed, nor financial status has any bearing as to who becomes affected—neither as the victim of the aging process, nor as the caregiver."

—Ariel Hernandez, Jr., M.D.

"My good friend Terry has provided us with a unique perspective as a Hispanic caring for her mother while living in another state. She reveals all her inner thoughts and feelings, which directed her decision-making. Others with similar circumstances will not feel alone after reading this story."

—Roger E. Arredondo, D.D.S., P.C.

"It is an inspiration to caregivers who want the best for our elderly loved ones and return the dedication they deserve."

—Jacqueline J. Stewart-Smalls
Owner, S&S Personal Care Home

"At the present time I am a caregiver for both my very elderly parents. This is a challenging responsibility and each day I come across individuals who like me have many questions. When I read Ms. Vasquez's book I found it moving and inspirational. In addition, it offered practical examples of how to deal with common issues of care. I could identify with her story. It gave me hope for my own journey. As the baby boomer population reaches their Golden Years there will be an even greater need for this type of information. I am grateful to Ms. Vasquez for this gift."

—Maria Antonietta Berriozabal
Community Activist/Consultant

"Terry Vasquez is a role model as a nurturing caretaker not only as a nurse but as a friend, mother, wife, grandmother, and certainly as a daughter. Being able to share her compassion and guidance as she cares for her beloved mother through her book is a public service."

—Antonio Tijerino
President and CEO
Hispanic Heritage Foundation

¡Mi Mamacita Tiene Alzheimer's!

¡Mi Mamacita Tiene Alzheimer's!

(My Beloved Mother Has Alzheimer's!)

Mary Theresa Vasquez, RN (Terry)

VANTAGE PRESS
New York

About the Front Cover Pictures

Left-side picture: This picture was taken about 1946. This is my mother, Mary Ruth Schultz, when she was in her mid-twenties, about twenty-six years old. Mrs. Schultz had three children by this time. She is wearing a shell necklace, which my father bought her upon his return from Hawaii where he was stationed during World War II.

Right-side picture: This is a current picture of my mother in November 2002. This picture is a copy, courtesy of the Texas Department of Human Services.

The opinions expressed herein are solely those of the author. The author and publisher strongly advise readers to consult with their own personal physicians and health care workers when deciding upon any course of medical or therapeutic program.

Published by Vantage Press, Inc.
419 Park Ave. South, New York, NY 10016

Manufactured in the United States of America
ISBN: 978-0-533-15724-2

Library of Congress Catalog Card No.: 2007900283

0 9 8 7 6 5 4 3 2 1

To *mi mamacita*
and all caregivers who care for a loved one
who has Alzheimer's

Thanks for caring Amor,
familia y
Fe, paso,
Jerry

Contents

Special Acknowledgment   xv
Acknowledgments   xvii
Introduction   xxiii

1. What Is Alzheimer's?
   (*¿Que Es Alzheimer's?*)   1
2. Why I Care for My Beloved Mother
   (*Porque Yo Cuido a Mi Mamacita*)   6
3. My Beloved Mother
   (*Mi Mamacita*)   18
4. My Preparation
   (*Mi Preparación*)   40
5. The Big Move
   (*La Gran Movida*)   44
6. Shopping
   (*Las Compras*)   48
7. The Day Has Arrived!
   (*¡Llegó el Día!*)   67
8. The Girl-Dog
   (*Cha-Cha-El Perro*)   71
9. Appointments
   (*Citas*)   76
10. The Daily Routine
    (*La Rutina*)   87
11. Activities
    (*Actividades*)   106

12. Training Day
    (***Día de Trainier***)   126
13. My Husband Visits Us!
    (***¡Nos Visita Mi Marido!***)   132
14. Taking Care of Oneself—
    Respite Care
    (***Cuidandose***)   140
15. My Sister, Liza, Visits Us!
    (***¡Mi Hermanita, Liza, Nos Visita!***)   150
16. Mamasitting
    (***Cuidando a Mamacita***)   154
17. Adult Day Care
    (***La Escuelita para Adultos***)   167
18. Special Occasions
    (***Ocasiónes Especiales***)   175
19. My Return to Washington   209
20. Epilogue   223

Appendix
    Favorite Mexican Sayings
    (***Dichos/Chistos***)   225
Bibliography   227
About the Author   229

Special Acknowledgment

To *mi marido,* Juan. *Gracias* . . . Thank you, thank you, thank you! Thank you for your love, strength, guidance, compassion, and patience of an angel. *Muchas gracias* for your endearing, never ending love for believing in me to accomplish the mission of caring for *Mi Mamacita con* Alzheimer's. ¡*Que Dios Te Bendigá*! (May God bless you!)

Acknowledgments

This book is dedicated to *mi mamacita* for being my mother! It is also dedicated to *all* the families and *caregivers* who care for a loved one who has Dementia/Alzheimer's. It does not matter what language one speaks or what culture one comes from, Alzheimer's does not discriminate, it strikes anyone!

First, I would like to say **Muchas Gracias** to my God for giving me guidance, strength and patience in order for me to take care of *mi mamacita* like a daughter, a caregiver, and a nurse.

Gracias to Jacqueline J. Stewart-Smalls, LVN and her Staff at S & S's CARE HOMES for caring for my mother as their own. *Gracias* to Clara Herrera, a friend of the family, for her tender loving care.

With all my love, hugs and kisses to my two sons and daughter in law, Jaime, Juan, and Alison. Of course, I will brag about my two sons, Juan and Jaime, who called me weekly and offered their emotional support. Juan also gave me a laptop computer so that I could complete my book while I was on the road. Also *gracias* to Jaime and his friends, Rachel Tyler Smoot and Steve Davis for their technical support. To my husband's current staff, Dave Rifkin and Jean Douglas, and former staff, Peggy Tabor, Amy Wei, and Javier Salinas, for their moral support.

There are no words in any language to say *gracias* to my younger siblings, Ray Anthony (Tony) Schultz and

Elizabeth Murphy (Liza), for all of their tender loving partnership in the care of our *mamacita*. They are 100%+ best sidekicks, honey-do's, rescuers, mama-sitters, photographer, dog sitter, seamstress, personal consultants, technical assistants, and many other talents that they bestowed on our *mamacita* and myself. They were there for our *mamacita! Gracias, gracias, gracias!* May God bless you and your families!!! *Gracias* to my sister-in-law, Diana Schultz, for her providing respite care.

Gracias to the following family members which include siblings, grandchildren, and great-grandchildren who helped with the care of our *mamacita*. They contributed and continue to contribute their love, money, flowers, cards, gifts, ran errands, bought groceries, visited and offered emotional support on a frequent basis to provide quality care for our *mamacita*: Sylvia Stillings, Robert and Debra Schultz, Juan and Alison Vasquez and their daughter, Claire Amelia and Maryn Graciela Vasquez, Jaime Vasquez, Ray Anthony (Tony) Sr. and Diana Schultz and their daughters, Kimberly and Heather, Elizabeth Murphy and her children, Carlos Quevedo, Valerie and Sarah Murphy, Debbie and Chris Larontonda, Don Carrington, Doreen and Michael Paradise, Jeff and Dr. Karen Monique Wuertz and their children, Nathan, Joshua, Jason, and Danielle, and Fred & Molly Kleitz and their children, Tina and Alex, Peter Burger Jr. and Gladys Burger and their daughter, Maggie.

OK, please bear with me; I am a Hispanic/Latina, so I need to thank everyone, including all my friends, *tías y tíos y médicos* (aunts, uncles, and doctors), and everyone else I might have forgotten! *Gracias* to our aunt Margaret Schultz for her loving care in visiting our mother. *Gracias* to Dr. Ariel Hernandez and Dr. Roger Arredondo for their professional medical and dental care.

Gracias to my mentor and friend, Belinda Arredondo, for her never ending moral support and wonderful suggestions throughout the whole process.

Gracias to my friend and Realtor, Diana Acevedo, who had the patience of a saint to show and help us buy our condominium in San Antonio, Texas for *mi mamacita* and I could live safely and comfortable.

Gracias to all my new Caregiver network friends that helped spread the word of my book, specifically, Maria Berriozabal. Alma Morales Riojas from MANA, A National Latina Association, and all my *comadres* from Las Comadres para los Americas, especially, Susan Santana and Carmen Lomellin from the Inter-American Commission of Women/Oas.

Gracias to all my friends who are helping me with autograph parties.

Gracias to the National Family Caregivers Association for their support.

Gracias to the Alzheimer's Association National Chapter, and specifically the San Antonio, Texas chapter staff, Hector Cordero and Tito Villalobos Moreno, the C.A.R.E. Advocates.

Gracias to the staff of Grace Place Day Care Center in San Antonio, Texas for their love and care of *mi mamacita*.

Gracias to the Department of Human Services for all of their contributions to ensure the elderly are taken care of properly and for the copyright courtesy for the front cover picture. Also, for my *mamacita's* interview which is located on their *2002 Annual Report* as well as their calendar. *Gracias* to photographer Eileen M. Llorente from the Texas Department of Human Services for my book's front cover picture.

Gracias to all my dear friends and neighbors for their

moral support, especially the Hon. Mary Ann Cohen and Billie Schneider and John Williams. Also thanks to all the new friends that I have not specifically named.

Gracias to Sharon Lewis, RN, PhD FAAN and the "Caregiver team" from the University of Texas Health Science System in San Antonio, Texas.

Gracias to my past employers and staff of the Hispanic Heritage Foundation, Inova VNA Home Health and my current employers and staff of the Inova Health System, HealthScource, who understood my mission and gave me the moral support to accomplish it.

Gracias to all my friends and organizations who endorsed my book:

- Sharon Lewis, RN, PhD, FAAN, Professor, Schools of Nursing and Medicine, The University of Texas Health Science Center, San Antonio, Texas and Clinical Nurse Scientist, Geriatric Research, Education, and Clinical Center, South Texas Veterans Health Care System.
- Belinda Arrendondo, Board Member, SALF, Board Member of Wolfe Trail Kids Kamp, Secondary Educator, Assistant Sales Consultant for National Publishing Company, San Antonio, Texas.
- Dr. Gloria G. Rodriguez, author, *Raising Nuestros Niños,* founder of AVANCE Family Support and Education Program, San Antonio, Texas.
- Rudy Valenzuela, FPS, MSN, RN, FNP-C, former President of The National Association of Hispanic Nurses, Washington, DC.
- Marisa Ramírez de Arellano, Chief Operating Officer, Hispanic Heritage Foun, Washington, DC
- Hon Carolyn M. Parr, Outreach Minister, Festival Church, Washington, DC.

- Pastor Jeff Wuertz, Chesapeake Community of Hope, Chesapeake, Virginia.
- Centro de Salud Familiar La Fe, Inc., Salvador Balcorta, M.S.S.W., L.M.S.W., Chief Executive Officer, El Paso, Texas and Juan H. Flores, MUP, Executive Director, San Antonio, Texas.
- The Family Doctor Office, P.A., Dr. Ariel Hernandez, Jr., San Antonio, Texas.
- Jacqueline J. Stewart-Smalls, LVN, owner, S& S Personal Care Home, San Antonio, Texas.
- Roger E. Arredondo, D.D.S., P.C., San Antonio, Texas.
- Maria Berriozabal, Community Activist-Consultant, San Antonio, Texas.

Gracias also to my other siblings, Carol Burger and her husband, Pete, Mary G. Roussin and her husband, Lynn, Pat Kleitz, and Ray Schultz and his wife, Betty, who were also available for our *mamacita.*

Gracias to the book *Getting Your Book Published for Dummies,* and its authors, Sarah Parsons Zackheim and Adrian Zackheim, for their guidance.

Gracias to all of the authors listed under *dichos.*

Gracias to my publishing company, Vantage Press, Inc., in having the faith and confidence and helping me to publish my book.

With everyone's help, I know in my heart I have accomplished my mission of caring for *mi mamacita* and I thank you! *¡Muchas Gracias y que Díos lo bendigán!*

Introduction

This is a memoir, a true story about a baby boomer daughter who devoted six months of her life to care for her beloved *mamacita* whom is Hispanic/Latina and has Alzheimer's. This story is unique because it is about a modern day baby boomer who moved across the country from the East Coast to South Texas to accomplish her mission in life; which was to ensure her mother was taken care of properly. As a result, the author left her husband behind in the Washington, DC area with the confidence of his love and support for their culture and family obligation. Her husband, in return, commuted to San Antonio, Texas every weekend to show his love and devotion to his wife and his mother-in-law.

The author talks candidly about the struggles, challenges and joys of a Hispanic/Latina family coping and living with a loved one who has Alzheimer's. This very personal story is written to emphasize the beauty of cherishing a loved one with Alzheimer's as long as one can. Each one of us is a gift from God. Caring for a loved one should be done for love, family and culture. The author tries to stress the importance of caring and encouraging the caregiver to do the best as possible with these situations. Alzheimer's patients are still very much human and need dignity and love as everyone. As per the Hispanic culture and probably in many other cultures, we were raised to care for our family (*familia*). As most of us know, if it is our calling/obligation, then we accept this obligation; no questions asked. This caring is done because it affects all of the family. We are a culture of family! (¡familia!)

This book is written in Tex/Mex style (with some Spanish/English words) because in the life of the author, as well as many other Mexican-Americans who live or grew up in South Texas, this is the language. As a result, some of the words go from one language to the other automatically, without any thought process involved on the part of the person speaking it; most specifically to other Hispanics.

Interestingly, this calling/obligation was given to the author upon her father's deathbed, or shall we say "death wish." Therefore, of course, the author accomplishes this calling with the help of God and family. Furthermore, this story is also trying to educate the Hispanic/Latino people and all the people who are given this calling/obligation of the importance of learning how to properly care for their loved ones with Alzheimer's. As Hispanic/Latino baby boomers, some too are faced with a new phenomenon of taking care of aging parents. The author wants to further emphasize that in the olden days, some Hispanics/Latinos were not given an opportunity to learn, and some struggled with lack of education because it was not readily available to them. I am sure that some readers have stories that have been encountered or that one's parents encountered.

Hispanics/Latinos now have an opportunity and obligation to learn, and the challenge must be accepted. One needs to learn as much as possible about Alzheimer's to take better care of oneself, our beloved parents and others who need us.

My book is *not* a reference book and is not intended to

be. It is, I would like to say, an encouragement and inspirational book. There are many wonderful reference books out there; I cannot tell you everything that I have learned about Alzheimer's within these past few years because there is a lot.

For good memories of my culture, I have placed some *dichos,* sayings, proverbs, throughout my book to make you smile and share them. I am sure that some of you were raised with dichos too; these dichos are very common in my Hispanic/Latino culture.

The suggestions given in this book are based on personal experiences that explain the qualities of faith, love, patience and family. Each person that has Alzheimer's is slightly different from the other because God made us that way!

Welcome to all of you who are caring for your loved one! Your payment will be in Heaven!

1
What Is Alzheimer's?
(¿*Que Es Alzheimer's?*)

Let us take a few minutes to talk about Alzheimer's. I guess I need to give an explanation about this disease to help one understand why and how I wrote this book. First of all, I want to say, I cannot, nor do I want to duplicate any of those wonderful reference books that are available. What I am really trying to tell is my true human interest story and motivate the reader to be better prepared to cope and understand, if the "calling" is given to them to care for their loved one.

What is Alzheimer's? (¿*Que es* Alzheimer's?) Now, that is a mouthful of a word! I am sure that some Hispanic people cannot even pronounce this word, much less understand what it is. As per the Alzheimer's Association literature, Alzheimer's is a disease that affects the brain and memory and with time, the memory is gone.[1] To be able to help a loved one with Alzheimer's, it is very important to recognize and report these symptoms to your physician *immediately* and for the thorough examinations which may include blood work and neurological exams. Symptoms (*symptomas*) may include:

Progressive Loss Of:
- of memory,
- of conversation,
- of ability to speak familiar words,
- doing daily chores,
- of recognizing where placed,
- of recognizing what is happening,
- remembering family,

Progressive Changes:
- of one's age,
- of one's personality and moods,
- of one's behaviors, actions, feelings and emotions,

Confusion and Disorientation In:
- Doing one's regular work,
- Doing one's daily routine,
- Making decisions,
- Communicating one's thoughts

Pérdida Progresiva:
de la memoria,
del hilo de la conversación,
del hable y del uso de palabras antes conocidas,
de las ganas de hacer sus actividades diarias,
de recorder donde ha puesto sus cosas,
en recordar lo que estaba haciendo recientemente,
de reconocer a su familia,

Cambios, Progresivos:
de su personalidad,
de su comportamiento,

de su comportamiento,

Cambios Progresivos:

Hacer su trabajo,

Cumplir con sus responsibilities diarias,
Al hacer sus decisiones,
En comunicar lo que está pensando.[1]

But let me tell you that Alzheimer's affects many, many elderly people. Just take a moment and ask around, your neighbor, your friends, everywhere. I am sure that they know of someone who has this disease. How awful! We even hear about it in the media and newspapers that Alzheimer's attacks celebrities; famous people as well as everyday people. Wow! It is something very ugly and frustrates a person because our beloved one has this disease. You all know what I am saying. It is around everywhere!

I will briefly share with you some of the latest information I have read from the Alzheimer's Association.[1] I further strongly encourage you to research for yourself because some of the studies indicate there might be a genetic risk of getting this disease. I personally feel that it is our responsibility to help ourselves and our family. Through my research, I learned this disease mostly attacks the elderly but on the other hand, it could attack a person as young as in the fifties. Oh, my goodness! (*¡Hay caramba!*) Not the fifties! Please, not me! That is too young! I also learned that it can last for about twenty years. More startling news is that presently, there are five million people in the United States who have Alzheimer's. . . . Now, that is a lot of people! More than 100,000 people die annually due to Alzheimer's.[1] Now, is that enough to scare anyone? What a terrible thing!

Ready for more startling information? Now, we are being told that the population is living longer and that includes Hispanics too, of course. That is a big difference, because the matter of fact is that these elderly people already have Alzheimer's. I can remember growing up and seeing my abuelita (grandmother) as well as many people in the neighborhood acting "strange." We thought it was a normal aging process growing old and being senile. As young children, we thought they were "crazy" (*locos*), but that was ok; it was acceptable because we thought that was normal. Another scary thing that I learned is that it might be in the genes![1] My grandmother had it and now

3

one of my aunts and one of my brothers has it too. Oh my goodness, I might get it too! Oh Jesus, help me! Not me! Today in this modern age, we have progressed in finding a name for it, but not a cure! Alleluia! Life is strange and puzzling! Wow! How sad! How scary! Oh God, please help us! How can this be? How are we going to cope? Oh God, please help us!

Here Are Some Mind-boggling Questions to Ask Yourself:

Do I have any questions? Do I want to learn more? Am I nervous? Am I scared? Did I give you a reality check? What treatments exist for Alzheimer's? How can one help our loved one with Alzheimer's? Which doctor do I call? What am I going to do? Is there someone who can be contacted for help? What about the checkbook? When can I talk with my parents about Durable Power of attorney? What is that? About DNR (Do Not Resuscitate), what about a nursing home if I change my mind? What can I do to help myself? Is there anybody out there? Hello, is there anybody out there to help? Is there anybody who can take care of my mother? Will I be able to handle this caregiver job? What am I going to do? I feel stressed! Questions, Questions, Questions! Yes, there is help! Thank goodness! Hurrah! You are not alone! You just have to ask!

- Do not worry so you can survive! (*No te apures, por que dures!*) (Author unknown)
- He who lives with hope dies happy. (*Quien con la esperanza vive, alegre muere*).[2]
- To have faith is the most important in life. (*Tener fe as mas importante de la vida*) (*Author unknown*)

4

Come on now, CALL the Alzheimer's Association, do not be embarrassed. They will guide and teach you to take care of your loved one, parent, grandparent (*padre or abuelito*) or significant one. 1-800-272-3900[1] Spanish is spoken (*Se Habla Español.*) Come on now! Call them! I called and they helped me and they can help you too!

I will conclude this chapter with some very special personal words I recently received from my younger sister, Liza, of what Alzheimer's means to her:

"Hi, thought I might write a few words down about mom. I know that Alzheimer's is viewed as a horrible thing to happen to us as we age, robbing us of memory and human dignity, leaving others to care for the basic needs of the individual. I have seen a lighter side of it. I grew up always looking for the silver lining even in the worst of situations. Maybe mom's forcing us to learn that religion paid off. All those forced summer CC DD's . . . for one thing, I shared caring for mom with a sister, which brought us closer together, forming a bond. Perhaps it was already there, and it was renewed and strengthened. As we grew older, some of us lost touch with each other, making new lives for ourselves, forming new families. I am glad I got the chance to share time with my sister in a very special way. Another thing I saw was that all the bad memories have been erased from Mom's brain. As a little girl, I knew she was unhappy, physically abused and treated like a prisoner, my dad being the disciplinarian. My mom worked hard, cooking, caring for many children. She now has a smile and no worries in the world. Her family has made sure that she will be properly taken care of until she is no longer here in the physical sense. I hope that once she passes, she will return our help from above! I am sure of it!"

2
Why I Care for My Beloved Mother (*Porque Yo Cuido a Mi Mamacita*)

First, things first, before I talk about *mi mamacita* and her Alzheimer's, I need to explain why I am taking care of her. Now that makes sense. One might ask, how was I, Terry, selected for this type of job? Let me reassure everyone, I did not ask for this responsibility. My father gave me this assignment before he died. I, like so many other Hispanics/Latinos strongly believe it is in our culture to care for our parents.[7]

In my younger days, I remember teasing my parents that the only reason they had a large family was to ensure that there would be someone to take care for them when they got old and sick. Now, that makes a lot of sense to me now. Guess what, they were correct! I also used to tease them that the only reason they wanted me to be a nurse was to take care of them. Well, they were correct there too! How smart my parents were! Presently, we, the children, have all grown up. We have all graduated from high school and most of us from college. Most of us are professionals and have better jobs than my parents. We are blessed that all of us are healthy and safe. I really have to congratulate my parents for the accomplishments of their children.

Gracias! Thank you Mom and Dad! It's my personal

belief that my siblings as *familia* (family), should forgive our parents for whatever wrongs they may have done in raising us because they did not know any better. They did not have parenting skills as we do today. But like I said, this is my very personal belief!

I am going to be sarcastic and say that it is payback time to care for my parents. I remember as a child, *mi mamacita* telling me and my siblings that we had to take care of her when she got to be a *viejita* (old lady). *Mi mamacita* also always told me that the world turns and we will find ourselves in the same situation. However, for everyone's information, this is not the only reason I am taking care of *mi mamacita*. I can just hear you say, here comes another one of those stories, once upon a time, a long time ago, *mi mamacita* said, "When I am *viejita*, remember who gave you *'che-che'* (breast-feed) and changed your *'ca-ca'* (pooh-pooh) diapers?" Come on, you can smile! All of you that were lucky to be breast-fed definitely will understand what I am trying to say, so smile and be happy with yourself. Have any of you heard of this same story? Is this story repeated throughout the Latino culture? Hmm. . . . I think yes!

- Respect your elders and youth will respect you.[2] (*Si, respecta a tu mayors, te respectan a los menores*)
- There is not time like the present.[2] (*No hay tiempo Como el presente*)

Please bear with me, just a little bit longer because, yes, I know this story is about *mi mamacita* but I still have to explain how my father selected me to be that special person. I am sure by now, one can conclude, I was selected because I am a nurse. Yes, you are correct, I

7

honestly believe that is the reason! On the other hand, I have to emphasize the person who cares for a loved one afflicted with Alzheimer's does *not* have to be a nurse or a health care professional. The only qualifications one must have is *faith, love, caring, patience and flexibility.* That's all! Come on now, you really can do it! Smile now and give yourself a big hug! My father had a lot of confidence in me throughout his life and called me many times about his health-related problems. He also called me about my mom and her "confused" state of mind. He did not know that she had Alzheimer's; that name was not around in those days. My parents had nine children. His job was to be our father. He was the bread earner and the disciplinarian of the family. My father treated each of his nine children the same; one could not question his decisions because he was our father. He was very macho and strict in everything. But I honestly feel he treated us individually. Even when he had grandchildren, he treated each person as his children and they did not escape the discipline either. I truly believe my father really loved *mi mamacita* but he showed his love differently and rarely due to his machismo. There were times in their lives that I feel that he did show his love for her as she once expressed to me. One of those rare times was during his military service when he was stationed at Pearl Harbor and World War II had just ended. Here is a copy of that special, romantic letter whereby he expressed his love for my mother and his children and his yearning to come home to Texas: (see next pages 9–11)

UNITED STATES NAVY

Tuesday
Oct 23 1945

Dearest Sweet heart:

Today I am writing you this letter to let you and darling babies know that I am well and pray to God you all are in the best of health, and doing fine, as these are my sincere good wishes of mine Darling. I have been in this damn place close to two weeks already, in fact two weeks ago I wrote you telling I was to leave the next day, I remember I had my things packed and I have had them ready ever since because I'm too confident of leaving any time, I guess by this time you are thinking some thing may have happened, but please do not worry sweet heart, as the only thing that's keeping me here is the same keeping everybody else here too, and that is transportation across the ocean to the good old States, ships come and go every day, but there's thousands of us ready to go, and also there is the army, Marines & coast guards, we all have to share the same navy ships, the real hold up is the damn idea of holding us the whole fleet of ships in the States to celebrate Navy Day, wait and see, after that, there will be enough ships to transport everybody more quickly. Some of the boys here in the same barracks with me that came the same day I came are leaving today at dinner time, almost half of us who came that day have left, with a little luck I may leave in the next draft or so, please

9

have confidence and faith in God that he will bring us together soon. Darling, I am very lonesome for your sweet letters, they bring me so much happiness that I feel we are very close together, reading all about the things Sonny does around the house every day, the things our daughters do and say, I can imagine how anxious they must be knowing their Daddy is coming home again, only wished I could tell you exactly the day I reach home but that all depends on the day I go aboard ship and the time we reach the states, Boy oh Boy! I can hardly believe its true, after all these months of absence there's no words that will explain exactly how much I long for your love, your sweet kisses that linger in my heart every day, life is not complete without the love, without every day life with our babies I miss their every day doings, every little thing they did or said, now that Rosary is going to school and most of all that we have a darling son whom we had longed for so many years and I still do not know as yet other than from his pictures and his life as you describe them to me in your sweet letters; Reina, no te impacientes que ya muy pronto estaré con uds, me paso los días rogándole a Dios que ese día or el siguiente salgo, y por eso no te escribo con la esperansa de darte las nuevas el día que sigue, pero el día se pasa y otro día y la misma cosa. Madre, el

se le hace dilación que no salgo de aquí, pero tengo
muchas esperanzas que muy pronto saldré, hoy mismo
llego el airplane carrier U.S. Saratoga, figúrate
que ya llevo un viaje a los estados y aquí está
otra vez, tengo esperanzas de irme en ella, salo el
viernes o el sábado y estoy muy seguro que nosotros
que quedamos aquí sigamos en salida, tamkien
hay otros barcos que están para salir pronto. Honey
I am holding this letter until tonight, it won't go out
until morning anyhow, so I thought I'll wait and
may be that I get word to if I am on Draft tomorrow, if I am I'll put a P.S. on top or on the back
of the pages telling you when I leave if I can find
out, just a hunch because I know we are the next
to go out now, hell most of the guys who came with
us here are gone, keep in mind about seeing me in the
depot, S.P. on my way to Camp Wallace, I think we will go
through S.A. I want to see you & babies then, wish I had
time to go to the house to see you but I am sure we will not
be allowed, the shore patrol will likely be on hand to
keep everybody from getting off the train, I know this
damn Mary, Honey, a daddy se le ase dilación, no sabes que
tanto te hecho menos, mis sueños son muy dulces pero yo pre-
fiero el que fueran realizados, nuestra felicidad con nuestros
hijos son mis mas sinceros deseos. Mil besitos muy lindos para
Sonny e hijos lindos y para tin tambien una abrazos muy apretados
y con todo el corazón que muy pronto yo te los dare en persona, mis
sinceros saludes para todos en casa, tu Mama y Papa y todo
los amistades que se acuerden de mi. Siempre tu adulto

Wow! What a romantic letter. . . . It makes my heart swell with emotion!

Let me tell you a little more about my father's medical problems to emphasize why I think he selected me to care for *mi mamacita*. The last time my father called me on the telephone was about three weeks before his last Thanksgiving Day. Please, let me sit down and take a deep breath because my father had been sick many, many times, but this phone call felt very different! As a daughter and a nurse, who lived far away, I had an "eerie, gut feeling" this was "the phone call." As a nurse, I tried to prepare myself for this day and I knew this call would come someday and here it was before me! Interestingly, this particular phone call came from the hospital. My Dad told the nursing staff to call me because he was not discharged. I spoke with the doctor who told me my father was terminal! The doctor further told me that *mi padre* was unsafe by himself because of his blindness and amputated leg. I then spoke with my father who expressed to me his wishes to die at his home. I told the doctor of my respect for my father's wishes and Discharge Planning was started immediately. I called my private family doctor and explained my father's wishes and medical condition. I asked him if he would take my father as a new patient. The doctor approved and accepted the care. I informed my father of the arrangements for his move home that same weekend.

Pardon me for a moment, I must backtrack to prepare myself for my visit to San Antonio, Texas to care for my father because this was not a scheduled visit. Before I went to San Antonio I had to prepare myself as a daughter/nurse but also physically, emotionally, as well as spiritually. Please try to understand that one can never fully prepare for a home death, especially of a loved one, especially of a parent! I have never had a family member die at home, and no one knows when a person is going to die. I prayed to *mi Dios* (my Lord) for strength and guidance because my father was dying. I went to my home health job and asked for guidance from Hospice. As part of my preparation, I was counseled and given paperwork. I also spoke with my husband, sons and some siblings and planned my trip to San Antonio; that same weekend, I flew home by myself. Upon my arrival, I got into a taxi and was driven to my father's house. I borrowed his car and went to the grocery store and bought some food that was high in protein, easy to eat and digest and bought high nutrition drinks. That same evening, I drove to the hospital and spoke to the doctor and the pharmacist and received the specific discharge orders. After my meetings, I drove my father to his house. There were no words between us on the drive to his house, which felt like a very long drive.

I lived with my father for about three weeks. Life with my father was spiritually rewarding. This was my very *last* personal time with my father. I now must explain *mi mamacita,* could not visit nor care for my father due to her dementia/Alzheimer's. She could not understand my father was dying. Within a week, my father became bed-bound. On the second week, my brother, Tony, called and asked if he could help. At that time, Tony was in the military and requested special permission. His arrival was a wonderful, welcome sight as well as a life-saver for me and our father. Upon his arrival, I explained the plan of care, which was to make our father as comfortable as possible as per the doctor's orders, and our father's wishes. Even though my father's condition was deteriorating, his spirits were good. My father was very much alert and aware of his surroundings until the very end.

On my father's last week of life, he took long naps which were very unusual of him. My father never took naps! He stopped eating and drank only sips of water and some ice chips. One day, he told me to call the family, the Thanksgiving party in his house was still on. Of course, I called; I always did whatever my father told me to do! My family did come to visit throughout the week but not *mi mamacita.*

On Thanksgiving week, my brother and I took turns caring for our father. Now, we are talking about a 24 hr/7 days a week job, and each of us rotated shifts to preserve our strength for each other and our father. On Tuesday, Thanksgiving week, my brother woke me up about three in the morning and said our father was talking in a foreign language. After opening my eyes, I quickly arose from my bed and ran to his bedside and sure enough, I heard a foreign language. I was stunned because he was asleep and talking at the same time. My brother and I looked at each other in astonishment because we could not understand him. We both concluded that it might be some sort of "spiritual trance." Within a short few minutes, before we could blink our eyes, our beloved father quickly stopped this trance. My brother and I stood frozen for a quick minute, looked at each other and prayed.

When daylight arrived, it was Wednesday, I prayed for strength and guidance to help me understand the previous night's events. As I was contemplating as to what I should do, I felt deep inside of me it was time to call *el padrecito* (a priest). But I was scared; I knew that my father was not a very religious person and he would get upset with me for even suggesting it. I can remember trembling and thinking how I was to approach him. But,

14

quietly, I thought to myself, I have faith and I have to help my father. I also knew there were a lot of problems in my father's life and I felt it was my responsibility to ask his permission; not only as a daughter and a nurse but also as a Christian. As I walked slowly toward my father, I trembled some more and prayed. I got my composure together and told him of the previous night's incident. As he listened, astonishingly, he did not talk. Timidly, I proceeded to ask for his permission to call a priest. To my surprise, after a moment of silence, he said YES! Amen, I thought! Thank you Jesus!

Later that morning, I called the church and that same day the priest came to the house and spoke to my father privately. After the *padrecito's* (priest's) visit, we were told we had a very proud and strong father! That afternoon, I noticed an unusual quietness in my father. It felt like there was a feeling of peacefulness about him which felt beautiful; my father had found peace with God!

On Thursday, Thanksgiving Day, ironically, it was my brother's shift again. That night, my brother woke me and said our father was asking for me. I hurriedly got out of bed and ran to his bedside. As I approached, my father said, **"Terry, what time is it?"** I said, "It is **3:30 A.M.**; it is late at night, go back to sleep." He then said, **"It is not time yet,"** and I said, "Yes, Dad, it is not time yet, it is time to go to sleep." I looked bewildered. I had no idea what he was talking about! To me, it was late at night; I was sleepy and tired, I could not understand what he was talking about. Without hesitation, we went back to sleep. At **5:30 A.M.**, my brother woke me again and told me that *nuestro padre* (our father) was asking for me. I quickly rose from my bed, ran to his bedside and said, "You called for me, Dad?" He answered, **"Yes, I called for you!**

What time is it?" I said, "It is **5:30** in the morning and everyone is asleep and you need to sleep yourself." To my amazement, he started giving me some orders: **"Terry, take care of my Las Vegas VIP card, Terry, take care of my checkbook, Terry, pay the bills, Terry, take care of your mother, Terry, call the doctor. Terry, did you hear what I said?"** and I said, "Yes, Daddy." As stunned as I was, I did as I was told, but I really was stunned! I stood frozen at that spot for awhile.

I called the doctor and told him what my father said. The doctor told me that my father was dying and to keep an eye on him and to call him of any other changes. After that phone call we all went to back to sleep, including my father.

At **7:30 A.M.**, my brother woke me up again! He shouted: "Terry, look at Dad!" This time, things were a lot different! Right in front of our eyes, our Dad's whole body was rotating in a circular pattern on his bed. In astonishment, my brother and I both stood frozen and looked at each other! I immediately told him of our responsibility to protect our father from falling off the bed and we placed chairs around it. I also told him that our father was dying and we could not disturb this spiritual event. My brother and I hugged, held hands and prayed together. This spiritual event lasted for about fifteen minutes but it seemed much longer. My brother and I shockingly stood frozen in time!

Suddenly, my father's body stopped rotating! Suddenly, his whole body was manually and physically lifted up into the air (about six inches from the bed). As my father's body was being lifted, he crossed his arms onto his chest. He opened his eyes and looked up into the heavens (the ceiling). He

stayed in that position for a few seconds (which felt like a lifetime). He closed his eyes, repositioned his arms back to his side and slowly his body was lowered back down to the bed and he breathed his last breath! As frozen and shocked that we were in our shoes, my brother and I looked at each other stunned and awed and said to each other, "Did you see what I saw?" "Is Dad dead?" and I said, "Yes!" We cried, hugged and prayed. After a few minutes we regained our composure and I examined my father and called the doctor, the police and *mi familia* (my family).

I must re-emphasize this is a **true** story and these events really happened even though they are hard to believe! Later that same day, my brother and I talked about this beautiful and shocking incident; we both thought we saw a "light" but we are not certain. One thing we are sure of, we both saw our father die and go through this very phenomenal, spiritual event in front of our eyes! We feel very blessed! ¡*Gracias a Dios*! (Thank you God!) Everyone now should truly understand why I have to take care of *mi mamacita*! I am really lucky and blessed! Many people have told me that this spiritual event is very rare and we are truly blessed. I honestly believe that God gives us messages in mysterious ways!

- Pray without stopping (Orrar sin parrar)
- God is the beginning (*Dios es el Principio*) (author unknown)

3

My Beloved Mother
(*Mi Mamacita*)

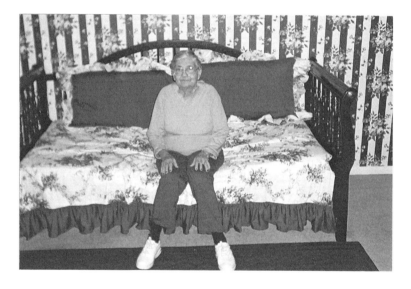

Mary Ruth Schultz

It is now time for the story of my beloved mother. I can almost guess that one is ready to say, it's about time one reads about this very famous mother (**Mi Mamacita**!) Of course, she is famous to **me** because she is my mother!

First, here is some background information. This is a

story of my mother who happens to be Mexican-American-Hispanic-Latina and also has Alzheimer's! (Please accept my apology and accept whatever title is politically correct to the reader.) It is about a daughter and her mother who live together under the same roof. It is the story of the challenges, love, struggles, daily activities of how I tried to enjoy *mi mamacita* and how God (*nuestro Dios*) lent her to me while she still smiled, laughed, continent and mobile. I took advantage of this opportunity and enjoyed her. This reminds me of a favorite saying, "Remember that physical or mental diminishment does not reduce a person emotionally or spiritually."[4] Like one of my favorite reference sayings (*dicho*) books said, "*It's all in the beans.*" ("*It's all in the Frijoles.*")[3]

I must confess, be careful when you pray for something, be prepared to receive what you wish for because there is a God (*Dios*), believe me, he heard me! My wishes came true, unbelievably! Oh yes, I prayed for the guidance in the proper care of my mom. I prayed for a sign to determine when to care for her on a full-time basis. I prayed! I prayed! Oh yea! I guess *mi mamacita* did raise an obedient daughter. I guess all those years of religion did pay off! *Mamacita* was right, as she was most of the time. After all, mothers are supposed to be correct. My God gave them the power to be correct! Now, all you *mamacitas* smile and give yourselves a hug!

Oh yes, my sweet *mamacita,* bless her heart (*su corazón*) and her brain, whatever is left of it. Through time, in front of my very own eyes, to my surprise, *mi mamacita's* brain was transformed from my mother to a child of about four or five years of age. I just could not believe it! In the early days, I asked myself, how can my mother, an eighty-seven-year-old Hispanic lady who weighs 120 lbs and is 5 foot tall, how can this happen? Oh, my goodness! This *mamacita* of mine, who gave birth to me and brought me into this world, now has childlike behavior. Can you believe she throws tantrums? Yea, real tantrums! I also have to smile and compliment her smiles which are beautiful sights to see; they just melt me.

Mi mamacita does have a good disposition and gets along with most people but not strangers. She is very scared of strangers. She has paranoia, and she gets very anxious when strangers are around. On the good side of her, she loves to be pampered. She loves to talk and can carry a conversation; it may not be relevant to today's conversation, but it is a conversation. Boy, does she love to talk! Here are some of her favorite words: "I want to go home, please take me to my home," and repeats this every five minutes. She also wants to eat about every one to two hours. I have to smile and share her two favorite sentences, which are like an old faded record, "I am hungry and take me home and I will pay you." One day, she told me that she was happy to have graduated from the second grade! WOW! Now, that is an accomplishment! Oh my goodness!

She also loves sayings (*dichos*). I am sure some of you grew up with these sayings and can remember them. They are part of our Hispanic/Latino culture, which have been passed down from generation to generation from one family to another. You may have already noticed some of these sayings throughout my book for pure reading enjoyment and good times reminders of parents and grandparents. Smile!

By the way, did I tell you that *mi mamacita* has a lot of energy? How did that point slip my mind? Sometimes, she outdoes me with energy, she does! The day care even told me Alzheimer's clients have energy like the "energy bunny."[5] The clients never get tired! However, beware; do not get on *mamacita's* wrong side! She might lash out with some cuss words. Oh yes, she says those Spanish cuss words that some Hispanic/Latinas grew up with. When I first heard them, I could not believe my ears. I said to myself, did she say what I thought she said? Hmm. . . . Once, I thought maybe I should put some soap in her mouth like she did to us children when we cussed but I changed my mind really fast. Smile! *Mi mamacita* cusses when she gets upset, anxious, tired and when she does not get her way. Of course, I cannot mention these words. Please do me the favor, sit down, close your eyes and think about cuss words (that you grew up with) and SMILE! You all know what I am talking about, those Spanish cuss words that are part of the Hispanic culture. Now, if you are a caregiver, SMILE BIGGER! Now, I cannot help myself, I just have to share her favorite line, please bear with me, she is so cute! Her favorite line is . . . Chin . . . ga . . . XXXX. SMILE! Another one is Pen . . . XXXXX. Hey mother, what words! One might ask, how does one cope? I had to learn rather quickly to ignore them and walk away until she stopped and also learned not to tire or get her anxious.

In the beginning of my adventure, I asked myself a lot of questions and went through a lot of emotions. What has happened to *mi mamacita*? Is she crazy? (Yes, I really did ask that question.) Why me? What did I do to deserve this life? What am I doing? Oh my goodness, what have I done? Oh my God, give me a break! Help me! One cannot imagine the emotions one goes through when a situation like this hits in the face, it is exhausting! At first, I was very exhausted and I asked myself, Why am I so tired but *mi mamacita* is not?

Please forgive me, but I must have some humor to help me survive this period of my life; for me to cope and be a better caregiver and daughter too. Sadly, I must say, it is now time to continue the true story of my mother's Alzheimer's. I will try to tell it chronologically to show how this disease progressed over a time span of about fifteen years or so. I would like to thank my dear Lord (*Dios*) for my mother's longevity. I first noticed she was getting forgetful about fifteen years ago. *Mi mamacita* was in the habit of writing a lot of checks to charities without my father's knowledge. I also noticed that she never balanced her checkbook. One day, I noticed that my father asked her how much money there was in the bank and she had a puzzled look. Surprisingly, this did not bother her when I or my Dad asked her. She just said, "I don't remember." Please note that this line takes on a special significance later on in her life as well as in her family. As time passed, *mi mamacita* herself noticed she was getting more forgetful and said to me that she was afraid of losing her checkbook. That day she also said, "Why am I forgetting?" One must understand that in the Hispanic culture, money and the checkbook are very sacred like in most cultures. In thinking back to those days, I have to thank *mi mamacita* for adding me to her bank account, and also for trusting some of family members to take her to an attorney to prepare the Durable Power of Attorney and her Will. In retrospect, I am glad this was done. I, as an obedient daughter, paid her bills. Let me tell you something interesting. One day, my mother told my sister Liza this story, "One never believes that the day will come when one grows old but, look at me now, I AM OLD." Ironically, *mi mamacita* knew she was getting old but did not know she was getting Alzheimer's! (After all, that was not a household word in those days.)

My people worked hard all their lives in their different kinds of jobs. Whatever job it was, it was hard labor and the money they earned had to be stretched to feed everybody. My father had two jobs, as most men did then, to make ends meet. That is the way it was. My parents had ten *niños* (children) but my mother lost a baby at childbirth so we grew up as nine. We were a typical large Hispanic/Latino family. *Mi mamacita* was responsible for the total care of all of the nine children plus three grandchildren. *Mi mamacita,* as most mothers in my culture, was also responsible for the children's religious education. Religion was accomplished either by attending Catholic school or through classes (*la doctrina*). Discipline was another responsibility she had as well as cooking, cleaning, ironing, mending and so forth and so on. In comparison to the women of today, they were a jack-of-trades. Some things do not change, as we know. Smile! In regards to cooking, of course, *mi mamacita* made delicious well-rounded tortillas, plenty of them! I remember very well *mi mamacita* making tortillas at all times of the day and night. *Mi mamacita* was always making tortillas. Every day as a matter of fact! Making tortillas was part of my Hispanic culture. Oh yea, now let me tell you about the art of making tortillas. Now, that is an art! I am sure that some of you can tell some stories about your *mamacita* and tortillas. I tried making tortillas but I could not master the art of their roundness. Oh how sad! My children and husband always joked that only *mi mamacita* could make real tortillas, so I gladly bestowed that job to my *mamacita*. Speaking about tortillas, my sister Liza and I were recently talking about our *mamacita* and our lives as children, she told me, "I remember sitting at the kitchen table, watching Mom roll out the tortillas every day. She had this really thick cutting board that she always used along with a rolling pin (*palote*). The ONLY thing is, I would watch her face and the expressions she would make while she was rolling them out. She would make all sorts of contortions, frowns, and looks that I was not familiar with. One day, I asked her why she made faces and she got upset at me (*me regaño*), 'DON'T LOOK AT ME,' she said. I think she worked out her frustrations out on those tortillas."

Oh boy, I do have to brag about *mi mamacita*! Of course, I will and you should too! She loved to cook! In those early days, everything was homemade. I can now say it was an art to cook for a large family. Some of my favorite foods that she cooked are fried potatoes, beans, enchiladas, rice, chicken, meat loaf, ranch-style beans, spaghetti, minced meat, chicken mole, bread pudding, banana pudding and roasted chicken. Shall I say more? (*papitas, frijoles, enchiladas, arroz, pollo,* meat loaf, *huevos rancheros, fideo, carne picada,* chicken mole, *capilotada y atole de banana*). *Hmm . . . sure smells good. Can you smell and taste the good food? I am sure that you can think of your favorite foods that your mamacita* cooked. Go ahead and dream on, you deserve to think and smell the roses, or shall I say the beans (*los frijoles*).[3] Bon appetite!

Mi mamacita was the typical Hispanic wife. She did everything that she was told to do by my father. She did everything around the house and ensured that all of the children were well behaved. She did the best that she could under the circumstances. In those days, my *mamacita* married young like most young women. She had her first child in her midteens. My mother did not receive a formal education; she received only a sixth grade education like many women of her time. *Mi mamacita* grew up in a large Hispanic family herself and I am sure that my grandparents and great grandparents received no formal education either. They did not have parenting classes in those days; they learned by example, good or bad, that is the way it was! My parents were not the best of parents but I have forgiven them. I must re-emphasize this point: I think that they thought they were doing the best they could; they did not know any different. In those days, some men were very MACHO and disrespectful of women's rights and children's dignities. I honestly believe they did not know they were wrong in their teachings and discipline of their children. I am not saying that it was correct which is NOT; what I am saying is I am sorry for what they have done to us children and must continue to live and learn from their terrible examples and not repeat history. I continue to pray to forgive them. I am happy that I have learned from their mistakes and have raised my sons with all the love that I did not have and I thank my Dear God (*Dios*).

Yes, I have forgiven my parents. I am happy that my father became a loving father before he died; he even told me that he loved me which he never told me before. During his last days, he reminded me often to call and care for *mi mamacita,* as I mentioned earlier. As for my mother, I too have forgiven her. I love her every day that I take care of her. In those days my mother had a lot of faith and that is what I think helped her cope with my father. She prayed daily and ensured that the children attend church and religion classes as I discussed earlier. We all attended church together like a family. Anyway, these are happy moments of my parents. Once they returned home, they each went to their separate households and my father called *mi mamacita* daily to remind her about her life's daily chores. My father even called *mi mamacita* on the day of his death. Now, that is love! (¡*Amor!*) My parents were separated for about ten years. Their separation occurred before Alzheimer's was a household word. Early on, she daily took the bus and visited my father and cooked for him and collected her one-half annuity. What a mom! My father, due to his blindness, could not drive nor travel alone so Mom came over to visit him. By the afternoon, she returned by bus to her parents' home. Like I said earlier, they had a love-hate relationship; we had no choice but to respect their situation. Ironically though, they appeared happier when they were separated. I think I need to explain about my parent's separation versus divorce. My parents like many Hispanic parents of those days, did not divorce even though they had their differences; they were both stubborn enough to stick it out for the children. I do have to thank my mother though for not separating nor divorcing. I do not know whether she was right or wrong but that does not matter now. She thought she was doing the best she could under the circumstances. They finally separated when all of the children got married or moved away from the house, and she moved to her parent's home.

Nine years later, in 1996, *mi mamacita*'s forgetfulness changed drastically; she suddenly stopped seeing my father. Ironically, she continued to ask for her annuity; way to go Mom! I found it amazing she remembered her annuity! Oh well! One day, *mi mamacita* told me she was aware of her forgetting things and was afraid of getting lost. As a result, I or another sibling picked up the annuity check and deposited it into the bank. Interestingly, sometimes when we spoke on the phone or visited, she answered the questions appropriately, but sometimes, she appeared to be somewhat lost. In one conversation she did not tell me the truth. In another incident, I noted she was afraid of leaving her house and kept her dog locked in. Furthermore, I noticed her house was beginning to show signs of neglect and I questioned her. She said, "I am fine, I want to live alone." My older sister and I visited weekly and helped her with the housework and the groceries.

Before my father died, I noticed my *mamacita*'s symptoms worsened. My mother's house was now very dirty! My mother looked filthy! It was obvious she had not bathed nor changed her clothes in I don't know how many days! I questioned her about her cleanliness and immediately she responded in an abrupt, sharp voice, "How do you know, you do not live with me!" How about that answer coming from one's mother? Boy, was I shocked! She told me off! There were other things I also noticed which included pieces of paper all over the house with written notes. Here is one example, which is obvious that a family member gave to her to write down her medicines as reminders:

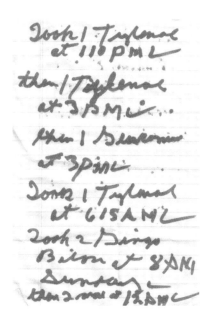

Please be prepared for the next few things that I am going to tell you and please forgive me. I am not telling you to scare you nor complain but I am alerting you of some of the symptoms of Alzheimer's and how awful and realistic they are! Another example: in the cabinets, I found money in different drawers as well as knotted, rolled-up tissue paper.

In her refrigerator, there was old, rotten food as well as dog food all placed together on the same shelves. Oh mother! (¡*Hay mamacita*!) Another interesting thing was the way she took care of her pets; she fed the dog and cats of the neighborhood about ten to twelve times per day. Anyone could see just by looking at the food bowls and also looking at mother's facial expressions, one could tell she was not even aware of reality. She was not even aware of the date or time but she was aware of her name and address. I also noted the stove was filthy, even though she did not cook. Upon further visiting her, she talked like she was aware she was forgetful, wondered why, and forget what she said. Interestingly enough, she denied anything was wrong and she mandated that she live independently. She told me that she did not want to bother anybody and this was her house and nobody was going to tell her how to live! Amen, I say to you Mother! It was awful; it was real scary for me and my family. Hey everybody, these are symptoms of Alzheimer's getting worse! It was extremely difficult and painful for me and my families to understand, accept and cope with these changes. It was also very difficult to help our *mamacita* because she would not let us. She would run us away when we came to help! I quickly thought, what has happened to my mother? She was not *mi mamacita* that I knew! What can we do? How can we help? I am sure that these same questions have come to a family member that is faced in this same situation. Amazing, how *mi mamacita* survived by herself! I think my God (nuestro Dios) took care of her! Amazing! Thank you God! (*¡Gracias a Dios!*) I left my mother's house with a desperate feeling in my throat and in my heart. I spoke with my husband, and several family members to try a find a plan to help our mother.

I tremble with fright to think how many people with Alzheimer's live alone because their families are not aware or refuse to accept the situation. There are some families out there in the world that do not care, too busy, too afraid to take responsibility or there just is no family! Now, that is sad and horrible!

Below is the family plan of care which I instituted:

First Personal Plan of Care
(Before Agency Was Hired)

- Take *mamacita* to the doctor for thorough examinations and medications as needed.
- Try to make a written plan of care: One must document, especially if one has a large family. Assign responsibilities if possible and ask for suggestions, whatever works in one's family because every patient and every family is different. However, remember, there must be <u>one</u> person ultimately responsible and the family must have respect for each other. This would be the best-case scenario but not a realistic one.
- In the beginning, one of my sisters volunteered and bought the groceries and washed the clothes. Since I moved out of state, I took care of *mi mamacita* on a long distance basis. My responsi-

bility was to coordinate *mamacita's* care. I ordered Meals on Wheels which provided proper nutrition. I called her twice a day to check on her status, reminded her about her medicines, her bath and change her clothes. I also paid all her bills and coordinated her medications, doctor visits and tried to ensure that *mi mamacita* was taken care of properly. I visited my mother about ten to twelve times a year to assess her needs.

- When my younger brother, Tony, got transferred from the military service to San Antonio, he, along with his wife, Diana (also a nurse) and their daughters, assisted with our mother's care.
- Tony and his family did the shopping, cleaning, washing clothes and weekly pre-poured the medicines in the pillbox containers.
- Tony visited weekly and performed all the "honey-do" around the yard and house.
- There were many chores to be done on the house because it was an old house and had no maintenance for awhile. He also coordinated the yard work with our other siblings.
- I encouraged all receipts to be saved. Believe me, it is tedious to do. (Nevertheless, reimbursement must be documented to prove to other family members and the courts if one is called to do so.)
- I kept my family abreast of our *mamacita's* progress through the e-mail and per the postal service. (Please bear in mind that this method worked fairly well for us.) Thank goodness for e-mail and cell phones. I tried my very best to keep everyone informed; it was a juggling act, keeping up with different changes in *mamacita's* life.

Please try to remember, coming from a large family or even a small one, everyone has his or her opinion. But one must respect one another's opinion for ultimately there should be only <u>one</u> person responsible for the care of a loved member with Alzheimer's.[6, 8, 9] We had many conversations about how to best care for our *mamacita* and we just could not come to a conclusion whereby everyone would be happy. I think the reasons are because we are a very large family, all professional, and all have varied opinions. That is life, I concluded! As one of my reference books says, "Since we know that many families in the United States today are tied to unhealthy patterns of relating, we can expect to find them entangled in the Alzheimer world too . . . siblings are likely to find all their old issues revived with unanswered needs and suppressed angers coming to the surface. A child who has seldom received nurturing care from a parent will find it harder than most people to become that parent's caregiver. Family members who have not learned to respect and cherish each other are not likely to treat the sick person with respect, appropriate attention and acceptance." [6, 7, 8, 9, 10] Like I said, that is life! Nevertheless, all the family is important and must help each other because it is very difficult taking care of a loved one with Alzheimer's.

After my father died, my mother's mental condition deteriorated some more. I bet that some of you might be asking, could this situation really get much worse? It is hard to explain but it did! Hmm . . . I wonder! I learned that in many other diseases, as well as Alzheimer's, a stress factor like death, may progress the disease process.[1] This, I honestly feel, is what happened to my *mamacita*. Nevertheless, she continued to demand independence. She would say, "Leave me alone, I am fine!" In response to her demands, I asked my family (*mi familia*)

31

to visit her more frequently. I continued to call *mi mama-cita* twice daily and visited every other month. There was one question that my younger brother and I kept asking ourselves frequently, "When do we step in and take care of our beloved mother on a full time basis?" I prayed for guidance and out of the clear blue sky, the answer came to me one morning like a bolt of lightning. I called my brother and said, "Brother, don't worry, there will be a sign and we will know. Whatever that sign is, we will know because it is our responsibility and *mamacita* nor we would have a choice." I recalled reading in some litera-ture, there would be a "sign." Believe it or not, the "**sign**" finally arrived ten months after my father died. On Sep-tember 16, 1999, my mother fell down from her bed to the floor. Ironically, this incident occurred during my visit and I happened to be outside of her house when I heard her shout for help. I immediately took *mi mamacita* to the doctor who said that my mother bruised her shoulder and he gave specific instructions not to leave *mi mamacita* alone and for someone to live with her on a 24/7 basis. Whew, I thought we were lucky that she did not have any broken bones! Thank you God! (¡*Gracias a Dios*!) From that day on for many years thereafter, *mi mamacita* con-tinued to complain about her shoulder injury. That night as I lay down to sleep in her bedroom, next to *mi mamacita,* I pondered as to how God works in mysterious ways. I said to myself, this was the "sign"; the "sign" that it was time to take over the full responsibility of caring for our *mamacita.* The next morning, I told my mother and family that I was going to take care of our mother on a full-time basis by hiring twenty-four hour care service at her home because the doctor ordered it. My mother was not happy with this announcement. She shouted at me to get out of her house and I did not know what was going on. I tried to calm her down with distractions and realized that no matter what I said, she could not understand. I decided to change the subject which seemed to work. I left her house concerned about *mamacita's* condition and at the same time challenged in her care.

My next job was to research by telephone, newspaper, neighbors and family to find a "live-in" lady. I looked in the newspaper want ads and the yellow pages of the phone book. I called my family, my aunt and friends. I e-mailed my family and told them about the doctor's orders and asked for their help. I made many phone calls. This project is very time consuming and one must consider the cost. I called the local chapter of the Alzheimer's Association and asked them for guidance and assistance. They mailed me information on their programs which she qualified for but they did not have 24/7 coverage which *mi mamacita* needed. I went back to the yellow pages and called agencies. I inquired about their prices, policies and procedures. I interviewed several agencies' sitters and hired one of them immediately.

I decided to stay home in Texas for about three weeks to ensure that the ladies worked out for my mother. At first, *mi mamacita* fought me, my brother as well as the sitters. She would say, "I do not need anybody else in my house." Please note she said these same words for about two weeks. I had to reassure the sitters of their job which was to help mother, clean her, clean the house, keep her company like a friend. After a month, I think my mother finally accepted that the ladies were going to stay! I do have to say though, that it took about three different ladies that tolerated her cuss words and her temper. Interesting note, I might add, I have several friends who also have parents with Alzheimer's and were going through the same situation of learning to cope with this very same kind of problem of parents demanding independence too. Very interesting! Here is a sample of the Plan of Care once the agency sitters were hired:

Second Personal Plan of Care
(After Agency Was Hired)

- Set verbal and written plan of care with agency for 24/7 sitters in my mother's house: One woman would come in from Monday-Friday, another one from Friday evening until Sunday evening. Sitters bathed my mother, cooked meals on weekends and ensured that Meals on Wheels were delivered during the week. Give my mother her medicines and ensured that medications were swallowed,
- Sitters would keep mother safe,
- Sitters would play with mother, watch TV, water the lawn and feed the dog,
- Call my brother for any emergencies, repairs, problems and questions,
- My brother visited weekly, brought groceries and picked up medications from the pharmacy, and pre-poured them into the medicine container. He performed any house repairs and mowed the lawn as needed,
- We both went to the bank and placed him on the checkbook. He would be responsible to write the checks to the agency,
- I was responsible to receive all of the bank statements, reconcile them and be responsible for all of the finances and pay all of the bills,

- My brother would call me for any/all emergencies, any questions or problems,
- I was responsible for regularly keeping our family informed of all changes in *mamacita*,
- My Aunt Margaret would continue to visit weekly if possible and inform me or my brother of any changes in our *mamacita*.

The next morning, I returned back to the Washington, D.C. area after I felt comfortable that maybe, just maybe, this plan of care for our *mamacita* was going to work! I received reports that my *mamacita* continued to shout and claim her independence, run off the ladies but they were instructed not to leave her alone at any time. At first, the agency sitters called my brother Tony about these complaints and he drove to our *mamacita's* house and try to calm her down. After about six months, *mamacita* finally calmed down and adjusted to the sitters. Alleluia! Miraculously, it was like a water faucet turned off! Boy, we sure were exhausted but were elated that she had finally accepted the sitters. Whew! Can you believe, the sitters became her friends and played games and watched television together.

About a month later, on a visit, my Aunt Margaret visited also and brought me a neighborhood newspaper want ad from another agency. I called them and discovered their rates were better, and I changed agencies. Mother seemed to have adjusted readily; I thought to myself, I guess mother did not know the difference, thank goodness! Being responsible for my mother's finances, I had to be diligent and research ways to cut costs because she did not qualify for Medicaid, Medicare or Social Security because, as I mentioned earlier, she did not work outside of her home. Her job was the care of the home and the children, that was her full-time job!

Caring for my mother at her home is my *very* personal choice; I could not put her into a nursing home because a long time ago, my *mamacita* told me not to put her away in a nursing home if she would ever be unable to care for herself. My, my, how my mother knew that this day would arrive. Hmmm. . . . Furthermore, I did not have the heart to do it. Besides, it was not in my Hispanic/Latino culture. However, to accomplish the adequate care of *mamacita,* I had to sell my parent's house, which was a very difficult task to do for me, but I had to for her 24/7 care.

After two-and-one-half years of my *mamacita*'s 24/7 agency care I noted that her bank account was dwindling out. I could not believe this could be another "sign" from God. One evening, I thought to myself, oh my gosh, not another "sign." That night, I tossed, turned and toiled as to the next decision I was to make. I spoke with my husband, sons and younger brother about the options. The conversation included asking the rest of the family (*familia*) for their financial assistance. I contacted them by e-mail (sample enclosed) and informed them of the situation. I received a few suggestions from some. Yes, I am embarrassed to say, I thought about a nursing home, some family members voiced it also but because I am stubborn and an obedient child, I could not live with this suggestion. That is OK if you decide to do this! The care of a parent is a personal decision. You and *only* you have to live with yourself and your decision but please research your options. If possible, pre-plan. It is much easier to think of your options without stress. Talk to other people who have gone through this situation. I called the San Antonio, Texas chapter of the Alzheimer's Association and I told them my decision of moving to Texas. I asked them for guidance and specifically, asked them for programs which were available. I was informed of a "Care Program" *mi mamacita* qualified and for me to call them as soon as I got situated in my new home in San Antonio. I was relieved and felt better that there is help through the Department of Aging and others! Whatever option you decide, it will be OK as long as you, the caregiver is OK! Swallow your pride! Do not be afraid! It is your responsibility!

Do well to those present and speak well of those absent. (Haz bien a los presentes y hable bien de los ausentes.)[2, 3]

Sample of E-mail to Mi Familia of My Moving to Texas: Mother's Care Link:

Dear family, I would first like to thank everyone who has helped Tony & me in caring for our MOM these past three years. It has been a most memorable, blessed and rewarding experience. I would also like to thank specifically Tony, for all his love, patience, dedication and endurance. He is a great brother, who is my partner, in caring for our MOM as per Dad's dying wishes. In addition, I would like to thank those family members that have sent in monetary donations, greeting cards, phone calls and visits to our mother. I would also share with everyone how lucky we are as a family to have each other. In addition, if I hurt anyone, I ask for his or her forgiveness. I never intentionally planned to hurt any of my brothers or sisters.

It has been over a month since I sent a letter informing family about our mother's dwindling finances in 2002.

I want to thank those family members that have responded and offered their suggestions and those who continue to send in donations. I have concluded that it is my legal and moral responsibility for Mom's care. As verbalized by Dad before his death, and as per Mom's wishes, I cannot put Mom into a nursing home. Due to the following reasons, I am moving to San Antonio in February to care for our MOM: (1) Mom's mental deteriorating condition, her financial status, her local doctor, her elderly age, other family members nearby, i.e. make her a loan to pay for the following until some money is received: (1) her groceries, (2) utilities, (3) security alarm, (4) round-trip flight cost to any family member to care for her in my absence including reimbursement to myself, (5) I will continue to fly with my husband for his work travels, (6) Mom will pay for the caregiver to replace me during my absence, (7) I will work part time as a Nurse to continue with my Nursing license, (8) I will sell her parent's home to continue to pay for her care. If any family member wishes to donate any money it would be greatly appreciated. May God bless each one of you! Please continue to pray for mom and myself. Please continue to call and send greeting cards to mom. Please continue to send money to me for OUR MOM. My best to all! Love, Terry

Oh well, this must be a "calling or a mission" that God (*Dios*) lined up for me all along and guess what, here it is now! What a surprise! What a surprise! Come on now, things happen! Those of us who are Hispanics grew up with faith that God does not give us something that could not be handled. Therefore, I said to myself, I must handle it the best I can, so be it; and of course, do not forget the husband and the family, they are important too! I do admit, after all, I am human! Many people told me what a difficult job it would be to take care of a loved one and of course I thought I knew better. After all, I am an educated professional, I am a Registered Nurse! I take care of senior citizens and clients with dementia and Alzheimer's. The **BIG** difference is that I **NEVER** took care of **MY** very own loved one. I also learned a very important concept that was not part of my Hispanic culture: one must take care of oneself <u>first</u> before one can take care of anyone else.[7]

To summarize, I have learned that living with *mi mamacita* on a daily basis is a very stressful juggling experience. I am sure many readers have multiple jobs outside the home as well as in the home and some also have children to care for too. Please try to remember, taking care of a parent is <u>not</u> something one should do without training, education and emotional stability. It is a different kind of job! It is a 360-degree reverse of the parent-child relationship. It is a role reversal. The caregiver becomes the parent and the parent becomes the child.[6, 8] Most of us have been raised to have faith and perseverance.

To complete this chapter, I would like to add other qualities to the word family: they are forgiveness, patience, trust, love, peace, and faith (*amor de familia y fe*). Like my husband says:

- Step on the gas (*Sume la bota*),
- We need guts (*Necitamos Ganas*),
- To do what is necessary is because of family and culture (*Para hacer lo que es necessario, es nuestra familia y cultura*). (*Credit goes to unknown authors on these sayings.*)

4

My Preparation
(*Mi Preparación*)

As I lived in the East Coast and *mi mamacita* lived in South Texas, I felt that I needed to find a place for both of us to live comfortably and safely. I could not live in her house, no way; it was very old and without the modern conveniences. It was built in 1921 and in disrepair. It needed new electrical wiring, air condition/heating and many, many other repairs. How did we ever grow up in those conditions, I wondered? I guess we did not know any better and our parents could not afford anything else. Most elderly Latino families live in very, very, very modest homes. However, their homes are their kingdom and rightly so! Remember the good old box fan or the window water cooler that provided "air" for the home? That was our A/C! Yea, it sure was! We just put some water in it and cool air came out for the HOT Texas weather! Wow! On the other hand, in the winter, we had the gas heater that sat on the floor. My parents turned it on with a match, a lighted newspaper from the oven burners. Amazing! Those were the times; we did not know any better! In addition, for keeping warm, my parents left the oven on at night. Amazing, my parents did not know any safety knowledge, nor shall I say, did they have any money or education to afford the comforts of a safe home.

WOW! How did we ever grow up and survive in those types of conditions? How times have changed for the better! Thank you Mom and Dad! In reflection, I do not think that I ever thanked my parents for raising me. In those days, we did not think that way! Maybe, we were not raised to thank them because it was their obligation. Now, as I have matured, I understand what my grandparents and parents tried to instill into us. It is now my responsibility to help my parents; it is in my culture and I have to make an example for my children and all our children, so they too can help when parents get old.

Now I took a deep breath and reviewed my decision to move. As I mentioned earlier in my family e-mail I feel that I need to elaborate a little more as to why I moved to San Antonio, Texas instead of moving *mamacita* to the East Coast. First and most important of all, is *mi mamacita's* doctor. Her doctor knows *mi mamacita* for many, many years. Secondly, she has some distant children in her beautiful, native San Antonio and I do not want to make a wrong decision. After all, San Antonio is where *mamacita* was born and that is what I still call home! Thirdly, everyone knows that the East Coast has real winter. I dare not risk her exposure to the cold, not if I could help it. I read some literature and some situations in my working experience, some elderly people cannot accommodate their bodies to drastic weather changes. Therefore, I was not going to accept the responsibility of *mi mamacita* getting sick. I thought to myself, move *mi Mamacita* to the East Coast and what if, what if, she catches pneumonia and dies? I would never forgive myself after all that we have been through! Silly me, how could I forget the real reason I did not move *mi mamacita* to the East Coast. It is my two-story house and all those stairs! How could I hear all her arthritic complaints and oh, her knees . . . can one imagine the many more complaints? Oh, mother! God bless her soul and her brain too!

To further prepare myself for my move, my husband and I flew to San Antonio during the fall to look for a condominium. To be honest, it was kind of fun, shopping. After all, this gave us an opportunity to buy us a second home, get ourselves ready for our retirement, and return to our beloved San Antonio. After looking at thirty or forty condominiums, it was exhausting! Thank God, the weather was cooperative! It took us about three to four trips to San Antonio to find the perfect condominium. Finally we found the perfect condo during the Christmas holidays. What a lucky *mamacita* I have! What a lucky daughter I am!

In looking for a condominium, here are some factors that are important:

- A gated community to prevent *mamacita* from walking out and getting lost,
- A first floor plan, with an adjacent bedroom,
- A large sized-locked patio for walking and exercise,
- Bright and cheerful rooms to stimulate her mind,
- A shower instead of a bathtub to assist with bathing,
- Close proximity to the doctor and the medical center,
- Close proximity to the grocery store and pharmacy and shopping! (Of course!)

After we bought the condominium, my husband and I flew back to Washington, D.C. and I continued to plan the move. I informed my three part-time jobs of my decision to resign because I was moving to South Texas.

I was fully immersed in learning how to care for my *mamacita.* I wanted to fully prepare myself for my move. I read literature and books on the care of the Alzheimer's patient from some of my nursing journals, the library, the Internet as well as the Alzheimer's Association. I felt that I had the obligation to learn all that I could to be a better daughter as well as a caregiver.

5

The Big Move
(*La Gran Movida*)

Finally, the day arrived; the day to move down to San Antonio, Texas for my new life with my beloved *mamacita*! It was one of those late January days which I remembered as I was growing up. The weather was not very cold in comparison to the weather in Washington, D.C. where it was cold, cold, cold! Thank goodness for the South Texas winter, I thought! Come to think of it, it was kind of stressful, my husband and I going to a different chapter of our lives, of living separately due to the ultimate sacrifice of the sandwich generation with an elderly parent. To help relieve the unknown stress of our new lives, my husband and I laughed a lot because reality had arrived! We both thought we were going through a comedy capers routine or something like that because the actual time had finally arrived and we had to pack. Can one believe, I am moving in the airplane! WOW! I frantically looked in my closet and toiled as to the decision of packing. After all, a South Texas winter was a lot different from the East Coast winter. In Texas, the cold spell lasts for only two to three days, but during that time, it is cold! BRRR, it may be as low as twenties one day and the next day, it is 70 degrees. Sometimes, the weather turns into spring and then summer all in the same week. That is our crazy Texas weather! Also all kinds of thoughts came into my mind; I was beginning to believe that this was not going to be an easy move. It was not going to be a piece of cake! Oh well! To top it off, I remembered airlines limited the amount of luggage. Finally, after several hours of packing and re-packing, I was packed, I think! It was funny to see my luggage. Wow! One would think that I was moving, well I was! Whew, barely made the mandatory number of luggage.

Finally, we both went to sleep about 1:30 A.M. At 4:30 A.M., this loud screeching noise comes out of the alarm clock. Ouch! What do you know, it is the alarm clock, I thought to myself. My husband and I tossed about the bed and tried to get a few extra winks of sleep, but knew we had to get up. As one can imagine, we were very tired; we were up all night packing. To top it off, we still had to drive one whole hour to the airport in Baltimore to catch a plane at 8 o'clock. Quietly, I thought to myself, we must *not* miss the airplane! As I fully awoke, I could feel butterflies in my empty stomach. Was it nerves, fatigue, hunger or what, I thought to myself? In my daze, my mind wondered off to the thought of, what if we miss the plane? How do I tell everyone that we missed the airplane? This interesting thought reminded me of a recent true story of the year we missed an airplane. Oh yes, we really did miss that airplane going to Colorado. It was one of those wonderful Christmas ski holiday trips with our sons and daughter-in-law. We were all excited to go skiing for Christmas. My husband and I overslept! Yep, we sure did! My husband claims that I gave him medication for his cold and, well, we just overslept! It sure was a nice, long sleep, I can honestly admit that. As a result, we had to drive to Colorado. Oh yea, we drove from Washington, D.C. to Brackenridge, Colorado! After all, we did not want our children to enjoy spending all our money and Christmas without us! Ha! Ha! The drive was an experience which has kept us laughing for a very long time. As a result of this, one can imagine that we were scared of oversleeping and missing the airplane again! Oh my goodness, we now have a history of oversleeping. NO, please (*por favor*) NO! Thinking back, I can say, how silly of us who were very nervous and bought two alarm clocks to ensure we would wake up on time and NOT miss this airplane! Amazing how silly we were and just laugh and smile!

Of course, we got to the airport on time and guess what, security here, security there, boy, what a day! Finally, the greatest day of my life, of moving to San Antonio, Texas to take care of my beautiful *mamacita* had arrived. I was now moving on to another chapter of my life, hurrah! But I kept thinking to myself the BIG question of how to tell *mi mamacita*. I had no doubt that I was making the right decision or if I could handle my new responsibilities. The question in my mind was, how and when do I tell my mother? I prayed and prayed for guidance and further thought to myself, I must get the courage to tell her but I do not know how. Of course, I got advice from many people and many answers; interesting though, there is no right answer. The answer comes from one's heart; I said to myself, if *Mamacita* does not understand, I have to understand because she has Alzheimer's and she cannot! Oh my goodness, what a situation I got myself into, oh, my goodness! (¡Hay, ya ya!) After several consultations with my husband, I concluded to be honest about my husband moving back to Washington, D.C. and ask her to move in with me. With this good feeling, I looked up into the heavens and placed my hands to my head in deep thought and said, "Dear Lord, please give me the patience and guidance, right now, please! Help me to take care of *mi mamacita!*"

- With patience you can win the impossible. (*Con paciencia se gana lo imposiblé.*) Author unknown.
- Everything willingly comes not to one who waits. (*A quell que esperar puede, todo a su tiempo y voluntad le viene.*)[2, 3]

6

Shopping
(*Las Compras*)

Before I picked up my beloved *mamacita* from her house and moved her to mine, I went shopping. I called my younger sister Lisa from Houston to come down to go shopping with me. I asked her to make a list of what she thought Mom needed and I did the same.

Below is part of my shopping list, please modify it for your loved one.

Please remember that each family is uniquely different. Below are some personal suggestions due to my personal experiences. BUT remember that each person is an individual, so please consult with your doctor FIRST—DO NOT SELF-MEDICATE! You MUST consult with the doctor beforehand in order to be prepared for any type of minor aches/pains that may occur!

For the medicine cabinet: (Para el cabinete de medicina)—Please ensure that the cabinet has a childproof lock!

Other medications:

- Vitamins (multiple)—easily swallowed, may need to crush, cut or liquid.

48

- Over the counter medicines for headache or minor generalized aches/pains.
- Over the counter antacid for minor stomach aches.
- Antibiotic ointments for minor skin scratches.
- Allergy medicine for allergy related injuries (cream, gel, spray or capsules).
- Anti-diarrhea medicine.
- Constipation medicine. Please be very careful because this is very common among the elderly. You may want to have available some raisins, peaches, juices, prune juice, high grain cereals or foods and drinking fluids. Be also conscious, the elderly get dehydrated easier. But remember to talk with the doctor first, because some people are on fluid restrictions.

Make sure and consult with the doctor FIRST before you buy. Educate yourself on the medications that your loved one is taking. Read the material that is given to you by the pharmacist. If you do not understand, call them when you get home. You must be alert that some of the prescribed medications cause constipation or side effects and know to recognize these and how to respond. Please be knowledgeable of what medications your loved ones are taking. They depend totally on the caregiver.

I must re-emphasize the importance of not self-medicating! Furthermore, I must stress the importance of consulting with the doctor before buying ANY over the counter products

Other supplies include:

- First Aid Kit (includes Band-Aids of various sizes).
- Thermometer—preferably a digital one.

- Ace bandage for the minor knee and ankle sprains.
- A scale—to check weight, for dehydration or over-eating. May need to weigh weekly or as directed by the doctor. This needs to be done early in the morning before breakfast at the same time each day or each week as directed by the doctor.
- Please keep a calendar/log report to the doctor during visits.
- Calendar to write appointments and important dates to remember.
- Writing tablet and pen available at each phone to write notes for the doctor.
- Please try to make a habit to write questions, notes or thoughts at the time that they occur.
- Telephone (with emergency numbers of: doctor, EMS, police, hospital and family members). Please write down the order to call **FIRST;** maybe a phone-tree system of each family member and who is designated to call whom.
- Emergency phone number (911), Doctor phone number; Pharmacy phone number (24-hour one as well as the regular pharmacy).
- Sectional/Weekly/Timed medicine containers.

<u>HERBS—DO NOT USE! IT IS EXTREMELY IMPORTANT THESE ARE NOT USED AND THAT THE DOCTOR IS CONSULTED ON ALL OF THE MEDICINES!</u> (*Yerbas-NO LAS USEN—<u>¡Es muy necesario que hablen con su medico</u>*!)

Safety checks—Make sure that ALL keys are hidden in a safe place!!

- Safety gates: for bedroom, bathroom and other rooms. (May use a bicycle bike lock to help secure patio gates),
- Child-proof locks for kitchen cabinet, stove handle covers and door handle covers,
- Check that furniture does not have sharp corners, if they do, pad them. Please note that the elderly may have sensitive skin and therefore may bruise and peels off easily,
- Slip-proof the carpet with commercial padding or if possible, remove the extra added carpet.

For loved one's bedroom—(*Para la recamada*):

- Plastic bed protector. (Keep an extra one on stand-by),
- Disinfectant solution and aerosol spray—(keep in a safe locked area and away from sight),
- Portable potty-chair (place a plastic underneath it if floor carpeted),
- For the bathroom, soft toilet tissue—(keep only one roll within sight),
- Television (hide the remote control),
- Large table lamp (they are very scared, especially at night; make sure that the lamp does not move),
- Safety child gates, (to place outside of bedroom),
- Slip-proof (non-skid) slippers. (Make sure they do **NOT** walk barefoot),
- Baby Monitor,
- Writing paper and pencil,

- Calendar,
- Telephone (with emergency numbers posted on the wall or attached to the telephone. These numbers are: of doctor, EMS, police, hospital, family members.

Clothes—(*Ropa*):

- Underwear, (a lot of them or disposable diapers),
- Bathrobe that has long sleeves, warm material, and with buttons,
- Pajamas—warm flannel kind with front buttons (to assist with warmth due to poor circulation),
- Blouses—long sleeve and with easy, large buttons,
- Slacks—(several) with elastic waistband.

For the bathroom—MUST LOCK (with child-proof lock—NOT with a KEY!):

- Safety bars in shower, slip-proof strippers or shower mat, adjustable shower head and shower chair,
- Adjustable side bars to the toilet,
- Hairbrush, comb, nail file and clippers—(**Lock!**)
- Toothbrush, toothpaste and mouthwash—(**Lock!**)
- Soap (very soft since they have sensitive skin and easily break down)—(**Lock!**)
- Body lotion (**Lock!**)
- Hair shampoo and conditioner (**Lock!**)
- Adult disposable diapers,
- Disposable gloves—lots of gloves! (**Lock!**)
- Soft toilet tissue (**Lock!**)

- Many various sized towels—(many towels, soft and various sizes),
- Dusting powder (for the body as well as the feet—they sweat a lot!—**Lock!**)
- Washing powder as well as clothes softener—(**Lock!**)

To play—*(Para juegar)*:

(**Remember, these may work one day and not the next. Also, this may work for only 5 minutes and then change to another game, whatever works!**)
<u>Toys</u>: very simple kind: (a) large pieced puzzles which have about 4–10 pieces, (b) coloring books (with large pictures, not too many pictures on the page—it frustrates them), (c) Large plastic markers (erasable), (d) Large playing cards, like ABC and numbers, (e) easy, adjustable toys, like for a toddler, i.e. blocks, (f) Try some animal videos (rent them first), (g) Try a musical book (rent first from library), (h) Children's books or magazines; try to rent from library or borrow from friends first, (i) a stuffed animal or a baby doll, try to borrow first, do **NOT** buy too many because they may not like them. **BE FLEXIBLE**!!! Minds are changed very often! **SAVE THE RECEIPTS**—P.S. I returned some toys because *mi mamacita* did not like them and several times I bought different kinds. You will learn what they like and dislike. **YOU HAVE TO BE FLEXIBLE!** Take a **deep breath** and **SMILE!** You must learn to **RELAX!** Take another deep breath! Think about something pleasant! Imagine being somewhere else having fun! SMILE and HUG (*abrazo*) yourself!

53

For the Kitchen—(*Para la Cocina*):

- Plastic ware, (spoons, forks, knives, plates, cups—NO GLASS, KNIVES, SCISSORS or any other type of sharp object),
- Fire extinguisher and written plan of exit—(posted somewhere visible). Do *not* forget to inform everyone in the house and your family who visit!
- Smoke and Carbon Dioxide Detectors (in bedroom also). Don't forget to replace batteries every year, preferably during Christmas or when the time changes. Set up a reminder system.
- House keys (may need to have a deadbolt lock or 2 locks, gate lock and maybe a chain/lock—(they WANDER about looking for comfort of their home when they were young),
- Food—they eat in small portions and many times. (They eat about every 2–3 hours,)
- Buy or cook food that is easy to refrigerate and freeze. Many have problems chewing. My mother loved to eat puddings, jello and fruit like bananas, and peaches, please be cautious with bananas because they may be constipating.

EMERGENCY—(*EMERGENCIA*):

In **advance, find** out from your nearest Fire Department the procedure for an emergency. Some cities offer the service **"File of Life."** This magnetic red packet contains a short questionnaire to fill. This way, when the emergency ambulance arrives, they will immediately read it and be familiar with your loved one. For example, name, diagnosis, anything in particular in regards to diagnosis, medications, allergies, physician's phone number and contact information. In addition, please contact the Alzheimer's Association and register in the *"Safe Return Program"* which is on a national database. The purpose of the program is to return your loved one home safely if he/she wanders off. As a means of identification, a bracelet or necklace will be provided and to be worn by your loved one.[1] I am sure that some of you have recently heard of some media reports whereby some people with Alzheimer's wandered off their homes; please note they were not on the **Safe Return Program.**[1] Do I need to say more? I do not think so! The Association also has other identification to show you being a caregiver.[1] Sample as follows:

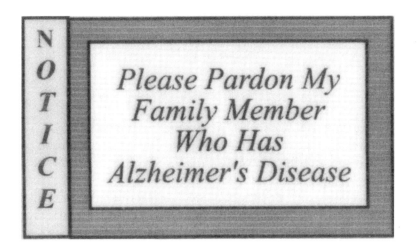

NOTICE

Please Pardon My Family Member Who Has Alzheimer's Disease

Here Are Some Other Personal Suggestions:

- Take your loved one to the doctor/clinic for their annual flu shot (usually given in October/December each year). If they cannot travel, you can arrange with your doctor to send a nurse through a home health agency.
- Take your loved one to the doctor for their pneumonia shot (once after 65 years of age or as indicated by your physician—please check with your doctor for specific circumstances).
- Take your loved one to the doctor at least annually and anytime that is necessary.
- On the first doctor's visit, ask for the procedure in requesting a disabled car plate/plaque so that you can park at a handicap spot. You might need to check with the Department of Transportation or the Department of Motor Vehicles in your city/state. (This might vary in each city/state.)
- Take your loved one to the Dentist at least twice a year.
- You might want to consider renting an emergency assistance service. This service will automatically send an ambulance, police if needed. For example, like Lifeline or something like that. Check with your doctor or the local phonebook.
- In advance, think about the decisions to make **before the mental/physical** condition deteriorates. For example, **DNR—DO NOT RESUSCITATE**, and feeding tube when not able to eat solids. These are not immediate decisions but need to be resolved **before** the situation arises and emotional stress sets in to the caregiver and to the family. Please speak with your family and be

prepared. If your loved one does not have a Living Will, Durable Power of Attorney and Will, check with a legal representative, an Attorney or the Department of Aging for the options which are available as per each state's requirements.

Additionally, before my actual move, my brother and I made a visual inspection of the condominium to ensure safety. Here are the Safety Adjustments my brother made:

- Installed safety bars and adjustable shower head on the shower bathroom/toilet.
- Child-proof all doors, cabinets, and stove.
- Checked and installed emergency equipment.
- Lowered the hot water heater temperature to below 120 degrees to prevent scalding (as per instructions on safety literature).
- Removed all solutions from sight and placed under a locked cabinet. (For example, detergent, soaps, etc.).
- Removed the life-size mirror in her bedroom (because she could not recognize herself and has paranoia).

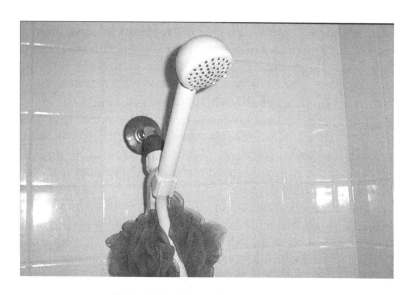

Adjustable shower head installed

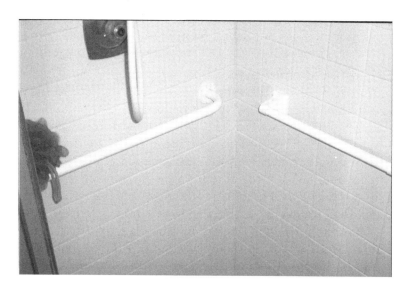

Shower safety bars

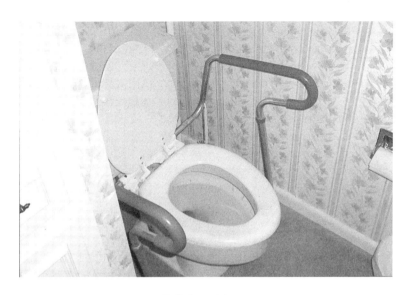

Toilet seat bars

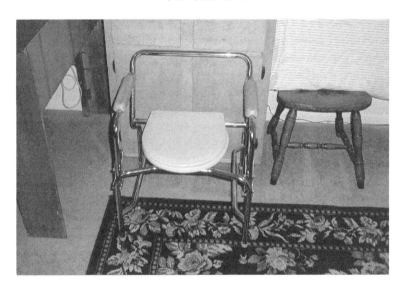

Portable potty chair

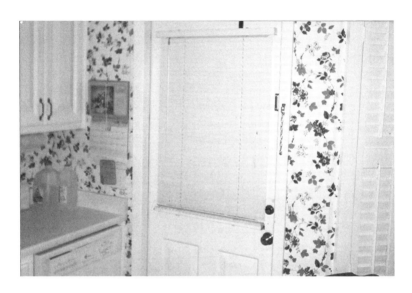

Door chain

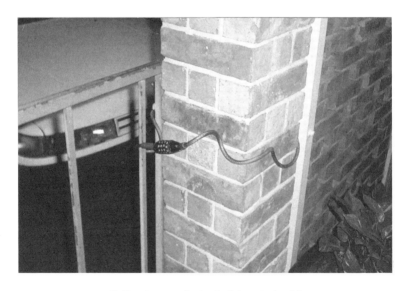

Patio door gate lock (bicycle lock)

60

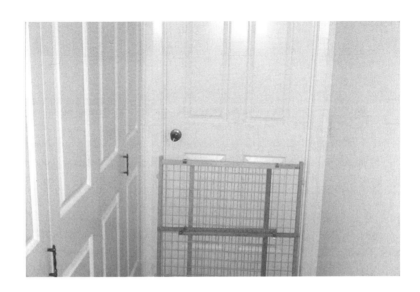

Safety gate

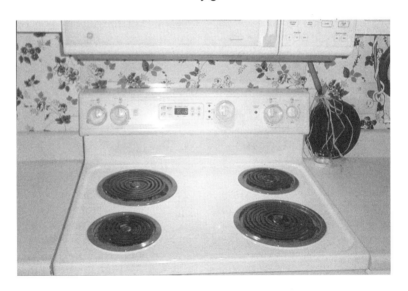

Oven knob locks and burner covers

61

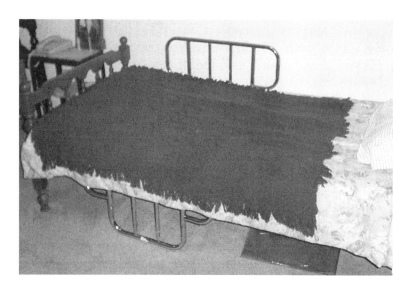

Safety bedside rails and plastic for accidental spillage

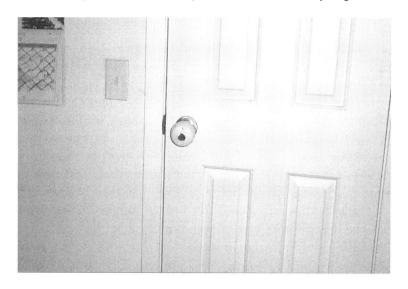

Door knob locks

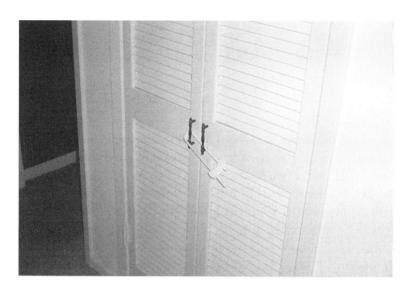

Hallway door locks

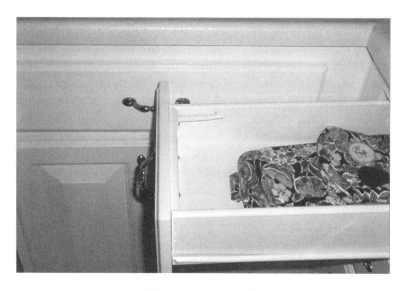

Kitchen drawer locks

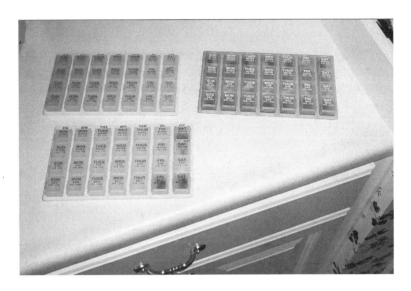

Secured medicines with containers and locks

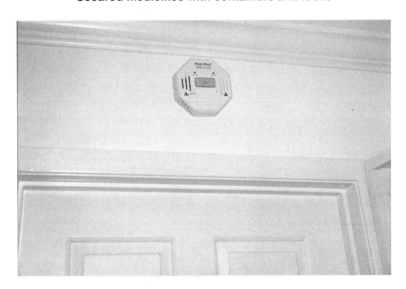

Carbon dioxide and fire detector

64

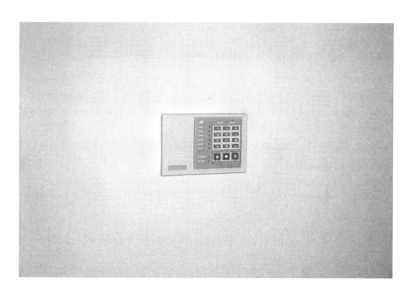

Reinstated emergency alarm

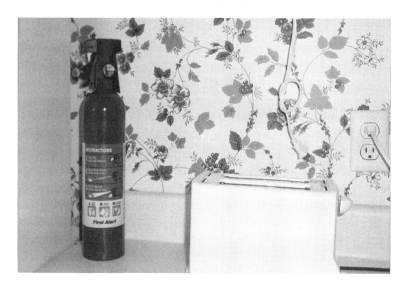

Placed fire extinguisher in the kitchen

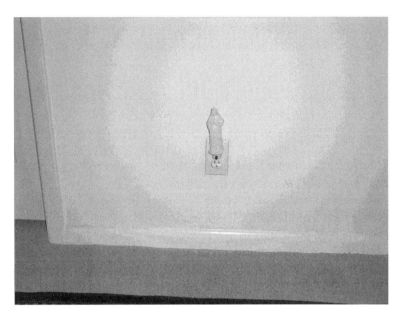

Applied night lights/lamps as necessary

7

The Day Has Arrived!
(¡Llegó el Día!)

The BIG day finally arrived and *mi mamacita* and I moved to the Northwest Side of town. Hurrah! I must explain our moving to the Northwest Side because as young children, we were taught the Northwest Side was a sign of progress. We all knew this part of town had more money, better education, etc. NO, it was not envy; it was just a fact! Moving to this area was a goal most people wished for and many could not achieve. Anyway, I was happy and so were my family members who helped us move! There was some fanfare, shall I say, family but no *Mariachis* like she had for her 82nd birthday! However, in my heart, I felt very content this day had finally arrived! The BIG day for my mother and I!

Before the move, my brother and I strategized the plan of action of the move our mother and her dog out of her home and into her new home "the condo." NO, trust me, the fun had not yet begun! We had to think and think and smile and think. This may sound somewhat silly and corny, which it was, but our goal was to convince our *mamacita* and at the same time, move all of her furniture. WOW! I thought to myself, what have I done? What have we done? I am not suggesting that the reader follow this plan, I am just explaining what worked for us. Whew! After several plans, we moved our mother and her dog to my brother's house. (We did this first so she could have her furniture moved out and she could not accuse us of stealing.)

Of course, we had plan B, C and D. And of course, we had to say a "therapeutic lie"[1] for the move could be accomplished. I took a deep breath and said, "*Mamacita,* you are going to visit Tony's family." She said, "OK." Hurrah, she believed me! Lucky me! Thanks to God! (¡*Gracias a Dios!*) Once she was gone from her house, I waited for the movers to help me. I was left alone to clean *mamacita's* house. Oh my gosh! Cleaning my mother's house was the hardest job I have ever had and at the same time the most exhilarating! It was a very difficult and exhausting job both physically and mentally. I went through each room and decided what to trash and what to move. I looked very carefully through every cabinet drawer, every corner, every newspaper and magazine because there was a family rumor my mother hid her money anywhere and everywhere. Of course, I thought to myself, wow, this could be a treasure chest hunt and I am all by myself! I laughed at myself thinking I might be a millionaire right at her house if I found the money. Unfortunately, after all my search, I did <u>NOT</u> find any money and I laughed again at the silly idea that she hid her money and that it was just a rumor after all. Hey family, there was NO money at mother's house, you all can rest your brains now!

On the other hand, though, I was very lucky because I encountered many memories of *mi mamacita,* her life and of my childhood days which was worth much more than any material money that could still be hidden in her home. One cannot imagine this tremendous task unless one goes through this type of experience. I laughed, smiled, cried and experienced some very deep emotions that are unforgettable which I will always hold dearly and deeply in my heart. This was a most overwhelming and exhilarating experience! I kept thinking to myself, *Where there is a will, there is a way (Querer es poder).*[2] I felt blessed!

Talk about flexibility, movers and family; funny thing, we thought that the moving plans were all worked out perfectly but the movers were late. You know family of course, what can I say, either they are sick, busy or late! What can I say, they are family! We love family, what is life without family? Life is full of obstacles I have learned. It is the way how one handles them that makes us mature. Life is a book and this one is another chapter of my life. I remember telling myself, I have to make a positive out of a negative in order for me to cope with this craziness.

Four hours later, the movers arrived with a truck. Hurrah! Well, about time! My brother, Tony, my husband and my nephew, Don arrived. Another decision we encountered was on what to pack and what to donate or sell. *Mi mamacita*'s furniture was old but not antique. Ironically, I did not have any more money or furniture, so *mamacita*'s furniture just had to do and we moved the furniture into the condominium. Later on, my little sister brought some of her furniture, plants and made curtains to make our house like a home. It sure was nice and homey.

Later that same evening, my younger brother brought our *mamacita* without the dog to our new house, the condominium. Upon her arrival, I welcomed her to my house and asked her if she would help me because I would be alone (that simple explanation was given to simplify her understanding). Most surprisingly, she said yes! I gave her a tour of the condominium as she smiled while we walked around. About fifteen minutes later, she said in a loud tone of voice, "Take me to my house." Oh my goodness, I thought, this new adventure was not going to be an easy one. Boy, was I in for the surprise of my life! I thought to myself, living 24/7 con *mi mamacita* was not going to be a picnic! Oh, my goodness! What have I done! I smiled, and closed my eyes and asked God for patience and guidance. I further thought of some *dichos* that *mi mamacita* told us as we were growing up:

Honor your elders and appreciate your young (Honra a tus mayors y aprecia a los menores),[2, 3]

Courteous words gain much at little cost (Cortesia de boca mucho consigue y nada cuesta)[2, 3] To those apt not to understand, few words are needed *(Al buen entendedor, pocas palabras),*[2, 3]

Do good and don't worry to whom (Haz el bien y no veas a quien).[2, 3]

8

The Girl-Dog
(*Cha-Cha-El Perro*)

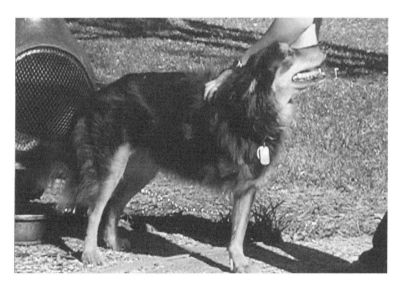

I feel that it is only proper to devote some time in my book
to *mi mamacita*'s dog because Cha-Cha (Girl) was her dog
during her Alzheimer's early phases. Cha-Cha, as she
was called, is translated into girl. She was named by *mi
hermanito,* Tony, because our mamacita did not give the
dog a name. Mother just called her Perro, which is translated into dog.

Lovingly, I will tell you about Cha-Cha. Cha-Cha is a collie. She is a beautiful black collie who has golden and white hair on her chest and legs. She weighs about fifty pounds. She is a lovable dog, a wonderful companion and protector of *mi mamacita*. Cha-Cha is the official welcome committee to anyone that came to visit. As soon as Cha-Cha heard any person at the gate, her ears perked up and would bark as a sign of people approaching. She, like most pets, got down on the ground or the floor and loved to be petted. She loves it and one can almost imagine a smile and a thank-you. I must brag to everyone what a unique, different dog Cha-Cha is. You see, Cha-Cha really is a different kind of dog. Cha-Cha is a three-legged dog and a sight to see! Miraculously, she really compensated for her handicap and gets around easily! One day to everyone's amazement, she jumped over the fence as she was running after a cat that apparently angered *mi mamacita*. Cha-Cha can do almost anything any dog can do. This handicap has not slowed Cha-Cha down at all! Anyway, so the story goes, as per *mi mamacita,* many, many years ago, *mamacita* found Cha-Cha on the side of the railroad tracks. Cha-Cha was just lying there on the ground apparently resting. *Mi mamacita* noticed that Cha-Cha was missing a leg and felt sorry for her. The story gets further complicated; I say this because one cannot substantiate what the truth really is. Anyway, *mamacita* told us that Cha-Cha had been run over by a train and nobody wanted her. She was left alone to die but apparently, she survived. Cha-Cha did not have any fresh injuries when *mamacita* found her. Cha-Cha was carried by my mother to her parents' home where she was living and automatically became the owner. Of course, we never dared to argue or question *mi mamacita* about Cha-Cha. It did not matter; Cha-Cha now belonged to her and that is all that mattered. It sure was a believable story in those days. Oh well, *mamacita* and Cha-Cha appeared happy. Cha-Cha lived with *mi mamacita* for about ten years, I think. When we visited, we all greeted Cha-Cha and played with her. We all noticed *mamacita* loved her dearly and treated her as her own child and overprotected her at times. About six years later, we all noted some shocking changes around the house and yard. When we visited, the dog food and the milk supplies were dwindling extremely fast. We also saw dog and cat food containers in several spots around the yard and house. There were also dog and cat feces in the house. What bothered my *familia* was that there were feces (uchy!) all over the place. We were concerned for *mi mamacita's* health. Amusingly, we saw the neighborhood cats come by and eat. It was quite a sight to see and it looked like they were having some kind of party. *Mamacita* did not appear to mind. It appeared these animals were her friends and she was taking care of them. On one of my visits, I saw *mi mamacita* would not let Cha-Cha go outdoors to play or do her private responsibility, and the sitters further confirmed this story. I questioned *mi mamacita* and she told me that she was afraid the dog-catchers would take Cha-Cha away. Another story that was told to me, was about *mi mamacita* not sleeping at night because she was always concerned about covering Cha-Cha with a blanket. Cha-Cha turned from side to side and there went the blanket too.

We were also most concerned for Cha-Cha's health. She needed flea baths, immunizations and bathroom privileges. Of course, we understood how important these animals were to our *mamacita,* but we noticed she could not take care of them by herself. We tried to get rid of some of the cats without success; they kept coming back.

In a sense, it was somewhat funny. One day, I took a cat to the animal shelter. To my surprise, the next day, *mi mamacita* had four cats to replace that one. I just smiled and laughed. It was obvious to us that our *mamacita* was the queen of the animals. As a result, a "dog plan" of care was established.

Our Plan

- My sister Lisa bought an indoor cat cleaner,
- My brother Tony was responsible for all of Cha-Cha's medical needs,
- Any other family who visited would clean the house,
- Once agency sitters were hired, they would clean the house daily.

Why Cha-Cha Was Not Moved to the Condominium?

The decision as to why Cha-Cha was not moved to my condominium with *mi mamacita* was solely mine! (Of course, I consulted with my husband and brother.) I prayed to my God (*Mi Dios*) for guidance and strength to help me make the right decision and it was made by my evaluation of our *mamacita*'s deteriorating mental health. *Mi hermanito* volunteered to care of Cha-Cha on a full-time basis at his home. (*Gracias!*)

I understand how important it is for the elderly to have pets. Animals are wonderful and faithful companions. Some of us have heard and read of the therapeutic value of pets. I agree 100% of their therapeutic value. I have personally seen this with some of the clients in my line of work. I too love pets. I grew up with pets, they were our friends. I even grew up with a duck and a lamb. My sons too grew up with pets. I would like to add my personal word of caution though. When a loved one has Alzheimer's, the pet may suffer. My *mamacita* was not aware of what she was doing. It is extremely important for the caregiver and family members to remember their responsibility; that is, the loved one and the pet's care.

Incidentally, since I moved my *mamacita* to her new home (my condominium) she has not asked about Cha-Cha (as I predicted). Whew! I was relieved! Say it is women's intuition or knowledge; I felt that *mamacita* would not remember. To this date, she has not asked about Cha-Cha. In passing, *mi mamacita* and I visited Cha-Cha and it was obvious to all of us that she did not recognize nor pat Cha-Cha. Thank you Lord (*Gracias a Dios*) for helping me make the right decision!

9

Appointments
(*Citas*)

As a nurse, a daughter and a caregiver, *mamacita's* health is of the utmost importance to me. I need to be alert and aware of her mental and physical condition for any changes that may arise at any time. So I decided to make appointments with all of her medical professionals: the doctor (*el doctor*), the dentist (*el dentista*), and the podiatrist, (*y el doctor de podriata*). **Please remember and tell the office scheduler that your parent or loved one has Alzheimer's Disease so that they can provide an evening appointment as well as limit the waiting time because of your loved one's limitations. These precautions will minimize any possible problems to all concerned. (One can try anyway!)**

The Doctor—(*El Médico o el Doctor*):

The first visit was a "getting to know" type of visit. I called and told the doctor that I had moved to San Antonio to take care of my mother. On the appointment day, the doctor and I spoke a little with my mother present; he examined her and asked her if she had any problems. As a matter of fact, my mother surprisingly said, "Why am I here? I am not sick!" The doctor and I both smiled at each other. The doctor and I then further discussed her medicines and her daily routine. My mother just smiled and did not say a word. She just stared and smiled at us. I told the doctor that *mi mamacita* was not sleeping properly and of her mood changes. The doctor gave me some prescriptions and they were filled at the adjacent drug store.

Two weeks later, I called the doctor because *mi mamacita* told me she had a terrible headache like "*me voy a morir*" (I am going to die). She alarmingly expressed, "I cannot see, I feel like I am going to die, I have a terrible headache." Of course, being a nurse, I thought of the worst-case scenario. Of course, I thought that *mi mamacita* was having a stroke right in front of my eyes. But, at the same time, there was something about her words and expressions that I could not put a finger on, she was not very convincing! Obviously, she was not in any distress. She was not even holding her head. Strange, I thought, hmmm. I knew for a fact *mi mamacita* always complained about her aches and pains because she has a very low pain tolerance. She is a chronic complainer and always had a headache ever since I can remember. However, this one was different, I thought to myself; she complained of having difficulty with her eyesight. Boy, was I scared! Of course, I could not show any signs of my concern nor panic. Interestingly, she kept staring at me and watching everything I did. One thing for sure, I did not want *mi mamacita* to have a stroke! As a nurse, I immediately but calmly took my stethoscope, blood pressure manometer and flashlight out of my nursing bag. I quickly examined her blood pressure, listened to her heart, examined her extremities for movement or lack of and looked at her eyes for any pupil changes. Surprisingly, during my exam, *mi mamacita* was very cool, calm, cooperative and smiled. After my examination, she did not complain of a headache anymore, to my relief. I concluded that everything was normal and breathed a sigh of relief. But, as a nurse, I could not take any chances. I immediately called her doctor and told him of mom's complaints and of her vital signs and we both concluded were in normal range. The doctor told me to take her in for a physical exam the next morning. For the remainder of the day, no more complaints of a headache were voiced by *mi mamacita*.

The next morning, I took my mother to the doctor and she did not complain anymore. The doctor examined *mi mamacita* which was normal. We spoke about the vital sign readings from the previous day, which were unchanged. The doctor then asked my mother about her headache, and *mi mamacita* said in a boastful voice that she never had a headache yesterday and never had a headache in her life! Interestingly enough, she was smiling and the doctor and I looked at each other and smiled too. Guess what, I thought to myself, I just had my first introduction to an adult tantrum! I had been made a fool of and I was being introduced to a different kind of life! I felt silly being at the doctor's office but it did not matter because my concern was *mi mamacita*'s health. I smiled in embarrassment. I felt that the doctor knew that I was only doing my best and I was not perfect. The Doctor just smiled and told me to go home and take care of *mi mamacita*. I then thought to myself, wow, living with a loved one with Alzheimer's is a daily learning experience. It is an adventure with many difficulties and many surprises. I strongly feel that each day is a blessing from my Lord.

Two months later, after *mi mamacita* entered Day

Care, she had another "tantrum" episode. I got a phone call that *mi mamacita* was bothering the other clients. I called the doctor, explained this situation, and medication adjustments were made. The doctor also cautioned me because of the side effects and to be extra cautious with *mi mamacita*. Within another week, the Day Care called me again. Yes, again! Medications were re-evaluated by the doctor and adjusted accordingly, again. Whew! I do have to confess I had a very good doctor for *mi mamacita* and he was always there for reassurance of my care and I thank him!

The Dentist—*(El Dentista)*:

As some of us know, some Hispanic people did not take care of their teeth. Maybe it could be due to the lack of money or because it was not very important to their health because of lack of education or it did not bother them until, a toothache actually arose. My mother is not much different either. I believe she probably went to the dentist many, many years ago but nobody in my family can remember when. One thing I do know is *mi mamacita* has only nine teeth and they look pretty rotten to me! She used to wear *placas* (dentures) but of course she lost them. She used to brush her teeth and lost the toothpaste and toothbrush too. She was lucky if she rinsed her mouth. One can imagine how her mouth looked. To say it nicely, uchy! We were lucky that she never had gingivitis or periodontal disease or something worse! I strongly feel that God has taken care of *mi mamacita*. Lucky lady!

Finally, the day arrived for a visit to the dentist. We both got in the car, buckled up and my cheerful mother asks, "Where are we going today?" I told her that we were going to see a friend, the dentist (he really is my friend). Upon arrival, the staff greeted us and escorted us to the examining room. *mi mamacita* and I were informed about the x-ray procedures. She smiled and was cooperative throughout the x-rays like a good little girl. I sure was glad of this. The dentist arrived and greeted us and introduced himself. He asked me for the purpose of the visit and how he could help. I told him that my goal was to preserve the remaining nine teeth that *mi mamacita* has and to prevent infection.

The dentist, through a show and tell session, discussed *mi mamacita*'s x-rays. He told us that *mi mamacita* had gingivitis and two bad fillings. (I was not surprised to say the least!) The dentist and I discussed the plan of care; this required frequent visits to take care of the gingivitis first, then the fillings would be taken care of. He gave *mi mamacita* an electric toothbrush and mouthwash and the hygienist showed *mi mamacita* and I how to use it properly. The dentist told us to make weekly appointments for the next few months. I was very impressed how patient and smiling *mi mamacita* was throughout this appointment.

For a few months, *mi mamacita* was seen by the dentist on a weekly visit to resolve the gingivits. After that, we made additional visits for cleaning and dental refilling. In retrospect, I have to share with you, these dental visits were a challenge and another learning experience for me. I was aware that *mi mamacita* required local anesthetic for cleaning and the fillings. I also knew that I had to learn time management in regards to the length of time that the local anesthetic would wear out and whereby she would be able to swallow liquids and solids again. I was challenged to learn of methods to help *mi mamacita* during these difficult times. Of course, *mi mamacita*, like many other Alzheimer's patients, loves to eat about every two hours. Believe me, they were not the best days of our lives together. Oh well, live and learn. What we did do, was to take drives, shopping, watched television, anything to distract. Also, I had available easy-to-chew foods and liquids as soon as anesthesia wore off. (I always carried these foods in my purse—BE PREPARED!!)

The big day arrived! The day for the fillings to be done! It was on a Tuesday afternoon, which most of her appointments were, to be able to coordinate the rest of her care better. I was somewhat apprehensive because I knew the local anesthesia took a longer time to dissipate because of her age. Much, much longer, I shall say. I was also apprehensive because I knew this dental trip was not going to be an easy one for *mi mamacita* nor me. Several additional thoughts came through my mind as I got myself ready and included the decayed fillings, the anesthesia and the pre-anesthesia medication. My mind went back to those dental x-rays and the decayed fillings which were pretty deep. To top it off, she had two of them. I thought to myself quietly, closed my eyes and prayed for strength for me and *mi mamacita*. I did not want to show any signs of my apprehension to *mi mamacita*. No way! At 1:45 P.M., as we walked together to the car, I told *mi mamacita* that today we were going to see my friend, the dentist. She was jolly as always because she loves to go for a drive no matter where to. Upon our arrival, the staff greeted us and guided us to the examining room. The dentist arrived, greeted us and we discussed and reviewed the plan of care. He asked how *mi mamacita* was doing and if we had any questions. *Mi mamacita* smiled and said, "No."

The dentist applied the local anesthesia as I held her

hands he proceeded to fill one tooth. Surprisingly he told us that this tooth needed only a partial fill. Alleluia! *Mi mamacita* did move a little and said, *"¡ya me canzo, vamonos!"* (I am tired, let's go!) I reassured her the dentist was almost finished. I also reassured her that she was doing very well and I was very proud of her. I told her that as soon as the dentist finished we would go "bye-bye" and she smiled. The dentist asked me if I wanted him to proceed to the second filling and I said, "Yes." The dentist proceeded to perform the second filling after confirming with the x-rays again. During his examination of my mother's tooth, he told me that this decayed filling was extremely deep and the decay touched a nerve. He verbalized his concern of the possibility of some unforeseen circumstance; if the nerve would be touched, extreme pain would result and could last for a long while. Ouch! The dentist further discussed this type of pain and the possible result of a root canal and pain pills. The dentist and I further discussed the options of preserving *mamacita*'s remaining nine teeth. He re-examined the x-rays and *mamacita*'s mouth again. I quickly closed my eyes and silently prayed to my God to guide me in this very difficult situation while I held my mother's hands, smiled and frequently reassured her. I quickly opened my eyes while I held *mi mamacita*'s hands for a sign of reassurance for her and me. The dentist then voiced his professional opinion to me. He recommended the complete removal of that tooth. I said, yes, remove it! Wow! I was so overwhelmed with the decision. I felt like a ton of rocks had been removed from me. At the same time, I was overwhelmed at the responsibility of protecting *mi mamacita* as her legal guardian, her nurse, her caregiver and most importantly, her daughter! This visit was quite a monumental one! Blessedly, *mi mamacita* did exceptionally well! Upon the completion of the procedure, the whole staff and I praised her for good behavior. *¡Gracias a Dios!* (Thank you, God!) Afterwards, as I promised *mi mamacita* and I went shopping. *Mi mamacita* now has eight pretty teeth which I am very proud of; I am sure she is too. You see, she loves to smile! Personally, I think she is proud of them too as she smiles bigger when I brush her teeth every night. Sometimes, I wonder if she is going to ask Santa Claus for her "two front teeth." It is okay to be funny and SMILE!

The Podiatrist—(*El Medico de Podiatra*):

Here I go again, making excuses for my people (*mi gente*). I want to take a quick moment and explain that the older generations of Latinos do not really go to the podiatrist; after all, what is a podiatrist? Some Latinos were not raised to go see a foot doctor, what is that? A foot doctor, what is a foot doctor? In the early days, a podiatrist was not even recognized by the Latinos nor a household name. The family doctor took care of everything! That is the way it was! My people have come a long way and they must also take care of their feet; after all, feet carry our bodies around, especially the elderly, diabetics and people with circulatory problems.

Yes, of course, I took *mi mamacita* to the family doctor so that he could trim *mi mamacita*'s toenails; after all, they had grown quite large. The doctor recommended I take her to the podiatrist, so I did.

I am going to try to explain how this appointment went because all appointments are very different. Here goes, I made an appointment with a podiatrist office by telephone through the receptionist; of course, that is procedure. I informed the receptionist that *mi mamacita* had

Alzheimer's and requested an evening appointment. The only appointment available was for about 4 P.M. I gave the receptionist all the insurance information. On the appointment day, we arrived sharply at 4 P.M. I did not want *mi mamacita* to wait too long. Of course, we all know, no matter how diligent one is in making medical appointments there is a waiting time. Well, of course, we had to wait! Thirty minutes had passed and I saw *mi mamacita* could not sit still any longer and she paced. I tried to distract her with her favorite books and a snack. She suddenly started pacing more and shouting to the other waiting patients that she was first. She also stared at them and me. It was obvious she was getting very anxious. She told me, "Look at them. Tell them not to do that." I tried to calm her down without success. All of the patients then stared at us in amazement. I approached the front desk, politely but upset, and told the receptionist that *mi mamacita* has Alzheimer's and we had been waiting over thirty minutes. I further told her that *mi mamacita* could not wait any longer. I asked the receptionist if she could please check on the length of time required for her present appointment. The receptionist said that we had to wait for the insurance company approval because they were from Washington, D.C. I further told her I had overheard her conversation with another patient also waiting for the insurance approval. (Ironically, *mi mamacita*'s insurance company was the same as the previous patient.) I reminded the receptionist that the Washington, D.C. insurance company was already closed because of the time zone difference. I was furious! I felt like telling her that she should have checked the insurance company earlier in the day or on the date of my original phone call (which was two weeks ago) NOT on the appointment time of an Alzheimer's patient! I further told her *mi mamacita* was past her patience and I was most assured the podiatrist would be reimbursed for the services if my mother would be seen NOW! I also told her that I would be happy to pay the podiatrist today. Coincidentally, the podiatrist was in the background and overheard my conversation. The podiatrist apologized, quickly guided us into her office and cared for *mi mamacita* most professionally.

Personal Experience

- When appointments need to be made for any doctor, dentist, podiatrist, please make sure and tell them that your loved one has Alzheimer's in order to minimize the waiting time (because these clients have no patience),
- Make sure to take a snack and drink if the wait/drive is long,
- Make sure to take a pencil/paper to write notes down. Talk with the appropriate doctor about the loved one's care and ensure that questions are answered. It is imperative that a good rapport is developed with the doctor, dentist or other professional. Remember that you will be calling and visiting them many times,
- I have made a practice to never alert *mi mamacita* of appointments too far in advance; actually I do not tell her until we arrive at the appointment desk because she does not understand and continues to repeat herself many, many, many times,
- Make the appointments at times that are convenient for you and your loved one; take into consideration their physical and mental situations as

well as their personal idiosyncrasies and of course the weather and driving conditions of the road. Do not be afraid to reschedule appointments due to car problems, weather or whatever the reason,

- Always be courteous; most offices are understanding.

10

The Daily Routine
(*La Rutina*)

I learned early on, a loved one with Alzheimer's needs a "routine." Interesting I thought, how familiar; we all need routines. Of course, that means my very own *mamacita* needs a routine too. As you read on, please notice my daily routine started on the night shift. Why the night, one might ask? That is because my first night con *mi mamacita* was the beginning of our new lives together.

Bedtime Stories—(*Estorias de la Noches*):

Our first night was somewhat cute. Here we are, *mi mamacita* and I in this big condominium. (Of course my husband is in the next room, shh . . . do not say this too loud!) Here I am, her daughter, and I am supposed to tell MY mother when to go to bed, HA! HA! I found out rather fast, the first night as well as the first few weeks were adjustments for both of us! Many adjustments if I may add! No matter how prepared one thinks one is, one never is! I read many books and had on the job training, and still it was not enough! A person needs both knowledge and training to accomplish any tough job in life! In retrospect, I have to smile as I write this book.

I must say again, this first night was the "turning chapter" of my life with *mi mamacita*. This gave me the opportunity to reminisce as to when I was a mother to my own children. It brought back memories of what I did and of how I went through a routine to get them ready for bedtime too. That famous first night, before I approached my beloved mother, I silently practiced to myself, "Hello, *mamacita,* it is time for bed." It is 7:30 P.M. I got the courage and approached my mother and noted she was yawning. HURRAH, I thought, she is sleepy already. Great, this is going to be easy, it looks like I too am going to sleep ALL NIGHT! HA! HA! Boy, was I in for a surprise! It is now time to explain the nightly routine! I gave *mi mamacita* her medicines and held hands and walked together to the bathroom to help her wash up. I reminded her to go to the potty; of course, I had to show her where the potty bowl was located. I also reminded her to flush the potty, wash her hands with soap and water and where the towel was located. I brushed her teeth, gave her mouthwash and showed her how to swish it around the mouth and spit it out because she had forgotten to do this basic care. She then said, "Uchy, that stuff is ugly." I complimented her of a job well done. Whew! I was pleased that job was accomplished. Onward to bed, we walked together to her bedroom. I said, "Mother, it is time to go to sleep." She smiled and said, "Are you going to sleep with me?" and I said, "Yes." I then put her pajamas on and I guided her to her bed. She sat down on her bed, smiled and observed me as I set the blankets for the night. I also prepared the bedside area for the night. I placed a plastic over the carpet and the potty-chair parallel to her bed. I also placed disinfectant in the potty bowl and placed a roll of toilet tissue on top of the potty-chair. I placed a trash can and wipies next to the potty-chair. Upon my completion of these duties I said, "*mamacita,* it is time to go to sleep, lie down on your bed." To my amazement she laid down on her bed. I put the side rails up and I covered her with a bedspread. I went to the extra bed across from hers and lay myself down. I started saying the nighttime prayers which she repeated. I kissed her and said, "Good night, Mother, have a good night." (*"Buenas noches, mamacita, hasta mañana"*). She said, "Good night, until tomorrow if God wants it." (*Buenas noches mija, hasta mañana, si Dios lo quierer*).

As I lay my head down to position myself on my bed, all of a sudden, within two minutes, *mi mamacita* shouted a loud verbal checklist: "Did you close the door? Did you turn off the light? Did you close the kitchen door? Someone is coming to kill us! Did you lock the door? I am scared! Did you lock the door?"

I have read and learned first-hand; loved ones with Alzheimer's have a lot of fear and paranoia and need a lot of tender loving care (TLC). Oh, yeah, I remember those initials from nursing school. Do not be embarrassed to hug, kiss and love them. They are afraid of the night, of people, of being killed or just about everything. They need a lot of reassurance.[1, 8] In my desperation and disbelief, I quickly covered my ears and looked stunned! She repeated this set of questions like a broken record for over ten minutes. I quickly thought to myself, I don't believe what is happening; it is going to be a rough and long night. A night I will never forget! Without second thoughts, I immediately got up, ran to her bedside and hugged her. I answered her questions each time that she repeated them again. I reassured her we were safe and God (*Dios*) was taking care of us. I further instructed her to pray and to have faith (*fe*). Quietly, I too, prayed that our God (*Dios*) would help *mamacita* go to sleep and give me patience to take care of her. I told her, "Go to sleep," I quickly went back to my bed and closed my eyes and pretended to be asleep. **FINALLY,** about thirty minutes later, she fell asleep. Amen! *Mi mamacita* is asleep!

Like a mouse, I gently tiptoed to her bed and ensured she was asleep. Whew, I said to myself, great, she is asleep! I ensured that the baby monitor was turned on, smiled with a big grin and slowly turned myself around and tiptoed out of her bedroom and into the adjacent bedroom to visit my husband. (Please note that some people are very sensitive to noise which includes *mi mamacita.*) I gently closed her door and placed the safety gate outside her doorway to ensure she does not wander and to protect her. I closed our bedroom door and ensured the second portion of the baby monitor was turned on. Whew! Finally, time with my husband! Hurrah! We both smiled. We talked of *mamacita*'s paranoia, the day's move and how we were going to adjust to our new lives with *mi mamacita.* We prayed together as we always do and finally we both went to sleep.

All of a sudden, we both heard some noise coming from the baby monitors. It sounded like water dripping. My husband and I looked at each other in astonishment and smiled. I arose from my bed to listen more carefully. Guess what? *Mi mamacita* was going to the bathroom in the potty-chair. Well, talk about privacy for *mi mamacita.* No way, *mamacita*, sorry about that! I listened attentively to make sure that she returned to her bed without any difficulty and she did. *Gracias a Dios* (Thanks to God). My husband and I looked at each other, smiled and chuckled, again I remember looking at the clock, which read 12:30 A.M. and I thought to myself, oh well. My husband and I immediately went back to sleep without difficulty. At about 2:30 A.M., the water noise woke us up again! Again, I listened attentively to ensure that *mi mamacita* returned to sleep and she did and so did we. At about 4:30 A.M., the water noise returned again! I listened again! This time, my husband and I looked at each other and shook our heads dazed and in amazement. By now, after being awoken about four times, I am sure that one can imagine how my husband and I must have felt. Oh, so sleepy and tired. I could see in my beloved husband's facial expression. I had to do something about this situation or else! Oh, so sleepy! It was most apparent he and I were not getting any sleep nor going to. I do have to say, in retrospect, these episodes reminded me of when my children woke us up during the night for whatever reason but not this one! Ha! Ha! After this water noise stopped, I decided to go to *mi mamacita*'s bedroom. I thought that maybe, just maybe, my husband could get some sleep. Of course, I too hoped to get some sleep; I wondered though if I would. I quietly tiptoed back to *mi mamacita*'s bedroom and sneaked to the other bed. I was relieved I did not wake her. Whew! I made it! I dozed to sleep almost instantly. Amen! Two hours later, to my surprise, but not really, I heard *mi mamacita* get out of her bed and I saw her walking to the potty-chair. She stopped and turned and saw me and said, "I want to go to the bathroom." I said, "Go ahead, the potty is there" and she proceeded to the potty. When she finished she returned to her bed without difficulty and immediately we both went back to sleep.

Believe it or not, daylight finally peeked into our windows. There were these big sun rays peeking through my window. I could not believe daylight was here already. Did the sun get my permission to come up I thought. Am I really ready to face the day? *Buenos dias* (Good morning) everyone! *Mi mamacita*, bright-eyed and bushy-tailed with a smile on her face, came to my bedside. I saw her approaching but pretended to be asleep. Oh, oh, how I longed for those few extra winks. Oh, how, I longed for sleep! She then spoke with a loud tone of voice and with a gusto of energy (*y con ganas*). She said, "I am hungry." Hungry, I thought to myself, does she know that I am very sleepy and tired? Does she know that she too was up all night? I thought, how can she be smiling and hungry? But all *mi mamacita* can say is that she is hungry. I could not believe my ears. There she was, standing in the middle of the room, smiling and waiting for food. After my composure, like a tired, silly daughter, I told her I was sleepy and to please wait five more minutes. I covered my face with my pillow and blanket and tried to go back to sleep. Ha! Ha! Less than five minutes later she said, "I am hungry, I am hungry, I want to eat." Amusingly, of course, I got up held her hand and walked her to the kitchen and sat her down and fixed her breakfast.

I quickly learned after two nights of this night time routine this was definitely going to be a ritual. Later this second morning, I called the doctor for help! I asked him to please order a sleeping pill for my mother; after that first sleeping pill, my mother slept like a baby. *Gracias*! Hurrah! I was so thrilled that the sleeping pill worked. Amen!

From that night forward and for a few month afterward, she continued to sleep some of the night, kind of, sort of. It is not perfect, but it is much better. Do not get me wrong, she still gets up to go to the potty, but not as many times. Hurrah! Thanks to the doctor and God (*Gracias al doctor y a Dios*).

Please sit down, smile and take a deep breath. Because it is time for more bedtime stories. Yes, please be patient and listen up. It is bedtime story time! I would love to share just a couple more favorite bedtime stories.

After all, they are uniquely different. I am sure that most people who care for a loved one with Alzheimer's have plenty of bedtime stories to tell too. So, please listen up. I will limit myself to a couple of them because, just because. They really are soooooooo interesting! SMILE!

There was this one "spooky" night. (Of course, this was before she was started on the sleeping pill.) I thought *mi mamacita* was asleep. How silly of me to think *mi mamacita* asleep! What a surprise I was in for! My husband and I are in the adjoining room doing some paperwork on the computer. Of course, the baby monitor is on and before long, we hear snores coming through the baby monitor which lasted a few minutes and we both smiled. All of sudden, and not even five minutes had passed, our bedroom door swings open! Guess who is at our bedroom door? *Mi mamacita, mi mamacita* smiling! She said, "Hello, I was looking for you." My face turned white as a ghost. My husband and I just looked at each other in total shock and it took me a few minutes to get my composure together. I said, "*Mamacita* what is wrong? What are you doing here?" She replied, "I was hot, I am scared." I hugged her and said, "How did you get here?" I quickly thought, how did she get here? There is a safety gate at her door. How did she do it? She smiled and said, "I just climbed over the fence," and proceeded to show me how she performed this procedure. I was so speechless! I thought to myself, after all this, my *mamacita*, is eighty-two years old, has arthritis and always complains of her inability to walk. Well, I'll be! Miracles never cease! I further thought, I am going to have to enroll her in some geriatric Olympics somewhere. WOW! She just outsmarted me! Me, her daughter! I further thought to myself, *mi mamacita*, like the character, "Houdini" or something like that, has some special power. I escorted her back to bed, gave her a hug/kiss and reassured her everything was OK. I covered her with the blanket and said, "*Buenas Noches*" (Good night). I closed her door, attached the safety fence and went back to my bedroom. My husband and I just laughed, smiled and wondered how did she do a thing like that? Miracles never cease, we said!

Ok, now, here comes the "special musical night," come on now, one more story. It was one of those nights, after finally falling asleep and being in "la la" land for about two hours, I heard singing and music coming through the baby monitor. "Splish-splash, I was taking a bath," etc. I laughed and cussed (just kidding) between my teeth, to my sister Liza because she is the youngest daughter of my family and has a very wonderful sense of humor. She has always given our *mamacita* fun things to help brighten her mood and assist with bath time. This particular "musical night" was of a bright pink stuffed rabbit which wore a bright red towel wrapped around its buttocks and sang and danced a bath routine when the "on" button, was pressed. She apparently turned it on and the music started playing. Finally, after about ten minutes, she turned it "off." Whew! My husband and I listened and laughed. I thought to myself, I dare not go into her room and disturb her. *No way José* (this is one of my *mamacita*'s favorite lines). I was so happy when *mi mamacita* finally went back to sleep. Of course, the next morning I hid that rabbit and called Liza to tell her about our musical night. We both had a therapeutic chuckle!

Okay, okay, just one more story. Yes, I know by now you might be saying, another story? What silliness! Please bear with me one more time, just one more bedtime story, please. Promise, this is the last one! I want to share with you these real life stories because I strongly feel that my family like yours is important and these are therapeutic.

After the same nightly routine, the morning finally arrives. Hold on there, you are probably wondering, where is the story; the night was routine she said. Yea, the night was routine, but wait a minute, the story is coming! Try to imagine the beautiful sunshine rays peeking through the window shutters and waking you up. Well, to my surprise, this really did happen. Wow! I thought, am I really waking up by myself? It sure is quiet around here. I looked at the clock by my bedside and it said 9 A.M. I continued to ask myself, how I did oversleep? Is my *mamacita* okay? I am now really getting concerned! After all, *mi mamacita* always gets up before 9 A.M. I continued to ask myself, how did I oversleep? Is my *mamacita* OK? I hurriedly tiptoed to *mi mamacita*'s bedroom. To my surprise, I was literally stopped in the middle of the hallway! Before my beautiful brown eyes, I saw the potty bucket sitting on the hallway side of the safety gate (outside of her bedroom door). I was stunned! It was sitting there like a message to me. Nothing was spilled, (thank goodness)! It was just sitting there! What could I say? Nothing, I thought, except to be happy nothing spilled and to accept this message, whatever the message was! Very strange, I thought. God sends messages in many different, strange ways! I decided to open *mi mamacita*'s door and to my surprise, she was sitting on the bed watching TV. She looked very innocent and radiant. When she saw me with the potty bucket in my hand, she had a large grin on her face and immediately said, "It was full." I said, "*Gracias*" (Thank you). All of these bedtime memories, I will never forget!

Here are my personal experiences as routines:

Personal Experiences

- Bought a baby monitor and placed it close to her bed with the other portion in my bedroom. (Remember that the Alzheimer's client has to be monitored 24 hours). If you happen to be lucky enough to have an adjacent bedroom and feel comfortable to sleep separately, then a baby monitor is a **must**,
- For nighttime bathroom facilities, I placed a plastic on the carpet to protect it, applied disinfectant in the potty-bowl and placed the chair parallel to the bed. I placed one roll of soft toilet tissue on top of the potty-chair,
- Placed the trash can close by (even though it might not be used),
- Have Wipies available (even though they might not be used),
- Monitored the sleeping medication carefully for effectiveness or any possible side effects. Call the doctor if any problems occurred. (Be aware that the elderly are extremely sensitive to medications and the dosage may need to be adjusted or discontinued completely.) One must be very cautious!
- Remember, the caregiver needs to get some sleep too. Forget naps, there is no such thing. What is a nap? (*¿Que es nap?*) (I thought that all children took a nap, but I think that my *mamacita* has bypassed the nap phase because she does not nap.) I was just pulling your leg! Oh well, I could not expect to have a nap at my regular job anyway, what am I thinking?

Daytime Routine

Is everyone ready for the wake-up call?? Wake-up call, what are you talking about? No, please, I do not need an alarm clock. What can I say; I never liked that loud sound anyway. What kind of place is this? No room service, no phone service, just my mother saying, *"tiengo hambre."* *Buenos días* (good morning), how are you? Just, *"tiengo hambre"* (I am hungry). Of course, I have to wake up, I have no choice!

Remember earlier, I mentioned of the importance of establishing a routine? Well, yes, a daytime routine is very important too. Around here, daylight comes to my little house a little early if I may add. Ready or not, *mi mamacita* seems to have an inner clock that tells her it is time to wake up to eat. As I mentioned before, this sure reminds me of the time when my boys were babies and toddlers. They too woke up with hunger. This sure is coincidental, I might add. Of course, I always tried to catch a few extra winks of sleep but it did not work; I wonder why not. How silly of me! Did I think I was on a vacation? No, way, José, as *mi mamacita* would say. If I didn't wake up right away, she paced the room for about two minutes and repeated, "I am hungry" with a great big smile on her face! I cannot resist this beautiful smile, so, I got out of bed. I usually said, *"Buenos días, Mamacita"* (Good morning, mother), and she said, *"Buenos días"* (Good morning). I grab her hand and we walked together to the bathroom. I feel very humble, being with *mi mamacita*. Routines consist of reminders: I tell her to go to the potty, wash hands, face and comb hair, and brush her teeth. These same reminders must be done many times throughout the day. I assign her to fix her bed while I take care of the potty-chair because I have noticed that she loves to help

97

with household chores. Some of these chores include, sweep, mop, wash dishes, fold clothes, anything! (They need to feel wanted). Remember, they still have their dignity and she is very sensitive to voice, touch and surroundings. She has an inner need to feel wanted and loved. She also senses if something is wrong, if I am angry or sad. Please speak slowly, look at them, give simple commands and speak clearly and to their face. Do not rush in your words. Show your loved one a lot of tender loving care, TLC. Hug them, kiss them, it is OK to show your love for them.

Try to understand that we all need love and understanding no matter how old or young we are. Yes! We all need love no matter who we are!

- A good deed is the best prayer (*Una Buena acción es la major oracíon*).[2, 3]
- "You may wish to express some gratitudes you've never actually spoken out loud before." [13]

Okay, we are done with loving; it is time to go to the kitchen to eat. Yup, let's go to the kitchen for "*papita*" (food). Once in the kitchen, I tell *Mamacita* to please sit down on her chair. I blush to tell you about her chair because it is a very special chair. It is a blue chair with a special hydraulic lift which automatically raises as a person stands up. I bought her this chair from a suggestion from her engineer son, Tony. He saw this in some magazine and felt that our *mamacita* needed it because of her arthritis. Interestingly, it works pretty good. I personally think this special chair is a pretty "cool" thing to have around. I must say, it is somewhat funny because the rest of the children will not sit on that chair because it is *mamacita*'s.

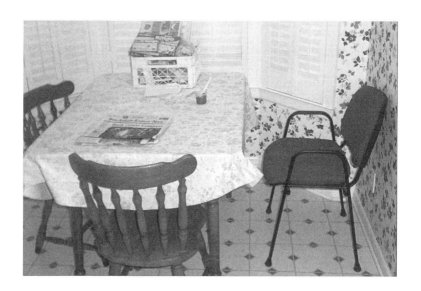

Finally, we are in the kitchen, of course; I am somewhat slow from lack of sleep. No need to worry though, I have no time to be slow. I am such a lucky girl to have *mi mamacita* to wake me up and keep me on my toes; never a dull moment, let me assure everyone! I would love to share with you her favorite words just in case you forgot what they are—"I am hungry." I have to chuckle to myself, of course. You can chuckle too.

Here Are Some Suggestions and My Personal Experiences

For meals: It is difficult to differentiate the times of each meal, but that is okay, *Mamacita* is always hungry. The routines I have developed, and really try to stick with, are as follows: (1) Make it a point to sit down in the kitchen three times a day for the main meals, (2) Sit down together as a family. Of course, yes, sometimes she eats my food and that is OK too. Remember, each meal must be in small amounts and nutritious because they love to eat many times. Do not forget to give them fluids even though they may refuse. But be aware if restriction is warranted by the doctor. Please try to remember they do not have concept of time nor nourishment.

- During all mealtimes: Please have available some toys on the kitchen table like dolls, books, colors, etc. to occupy *Mamacita* while I'm cooking.
- Cook small nourishing meals. Remember, they eat in very small portions. They eat several times a day; like 6–8 times/day. Be cautious; they have sensitive taste buds to temperature and texture. Examples: **for breakfast:** oatmeal or malt-o-meal, (1/2 pkg), pancakes or French toast (1 slice), 1/2 cup warm milk, 1/2 banana, 1/2 apple or peach, Jello or pudding. Try not to give too many sweets or café (coffee), **for lunch:** half of sandwich. Easy to chew food, like chicken, peanut butter, fish, minced meat like meatloaf, spaghetti, macaroni and cheese, thickened soups; liquids and snacks as above, **for dinner:** Easy to chew food—same as lunch. ¡*Buena Suerta*! (Good luck!)

Medicine Times—(*Tiempo de Medicinas*):

After every meal, her usual comment was, what do we do now? I told her, "It is time for medicines." (It is time to give *mi mamacita* her medicines at the designated times as per the doctor's orders.) Let me tell you most of the time she was cooperative but sometimes she was not. When she was not, I bribed her or told her a "therapeutic lie"[1] or a "white lie" so that she would take her medicines. "White lies" are interesting because they have been around a very long time. I was surprised to learn this approved technique to convince a loved one to take their medicines. I remember "white lies" from when I was a child. I am sure that you also can remember some "white lies" too. Smile!

Ok, here goes, true confessions, some "white lies" that I have told *mi mamacita*. Remember, to speak in a soft, firm and convincing voice with soothing facial expressions. NO SMILES! Please do not threaten or mislead them. They have "special powers"; they will sense that you are not saying the truth. Oh, so scary. . . . Here goes,

- "*Mamacita,* as soon as you take your *medicinas* (medicines), you and I are going bye-bye" (going out). Most of the time she smiled and did take her medicines. By the way, this is her favorite line because *mi mamacita* loves to go out for drives. As soon as you take your *medicina* (medicine), I will give you ice cream. Did I say ice cream? Yea, I sure did. Of course, *mamacita* took her medicines, and she loved to eat ice cream or any kind of food!
- "Can you please take your *medicina* because I have so much work to do and I need your help."
- "Please take your medicine and your arthritis or headache will go away." Of course, I never left the pills on the table; I gave them to her one at a time and stood in front of her. **NEVER** leave medicines alone in front of her without your presence; one must ensure that medicines are taken as pre-

101

scribed. I do have to tell you though, sometimes these white lies do not work. If they didn't work, I just walked away for 2–3 minutes and tried again. When I returned, she had forgotten the incident and did take her medicines. Funny thing, when this occurred, I was happy that she was forgetful.

Bath Time—(*El Baño*):

Afraid of the water and lack of bathing is a very common problem. The Alzheimer's person has no memory of cleanliness or lack of it. "Get organized" as my little sister advised me! I could not believe that I was getting advice from my younger sister, to me, her big sister. My younger sister, Liza, has raised seven children so she knows about organization. She is an expert! Therefore, I have no doubt that she could help me raise my "new five-year-old daughter," our *mamacita*. It would be a piece of cake for her because she is a professional domestic engineer. With an embarrassed smile, I confess, my younger sister is absolutely correct! "Get organized," as she told me! I foolishly admit that I felt I could handle this kind of problem. After all, it is only a bath. I thought how difficult would it be to convince *mi mamacita* about a bath? Yes, I was aware she was afraid of the water, but I had to "see it to believe it" with my own eyes. Oh, yea. Believe it! After one struggle *con mi mamacita* in the shower, that was enough and convincing for me! Convincing to me though, not her! She yelled and cussed at me and I could not believe *mi mamacita* had such a dirty mouth. I honestly felt like putting a soap bar in her mouth like she did to some of my younger siblings when we were kids. But I dared not irritate her any more, if you know what I mean. I really knew those bad words were not directed at me, but at the water. She was not in control, someone else was. It did not hurt me what she was saying because I understood. Nevertheless, I had to find the solution to this problem. I was challenged to find the solution as soon as possible (ASAP), like right now! I prayed and sang as a distraction and hurried as fast as I could; it helped some. She even accused me of trying to freeze her, and in a loud tone of voice, said, "Hey woman, I am cold." She also accused me of putting water on her. Can anyone imagine water on the body? Boy, what a surprise, my *mamacita* sure was a different person in the shower. Wow! It was so amazing! It was as if I turned on a switch in her brain which said, GET ME OUT OF THIS WATER! NOW! NOW! I vividly recall my ears still hurt from that first incident. Amazingly, that first bath was the fastest bath I have ever given! My 101-nursing professor would be proud of me. Smile now! After that bath, she was such a different person, like day and night, and she was nice as she could be. To this date, we have not spoken about this incident and I know it will be our best kept secret. Ha! Ha! Anyway, I am lucky that she has forgotten, thank goodness. That night, of course, I did MORE research on this special problem. The next day, I called the Alzheimer's association hot-line and the day care for advice.[1, 4, 8, 10] Bath times are different now; I am organized, faster, pray and sing more. I also take deep breaths, smile, and try to distract her with conversation; if she is ugly, I ignore her and pray/sing. She still complains, "Oh, I am getting wet, Oh, I am cold," but she is somewhat more cooperative, sometimes. My personal theory is whatever works for the caregiver, which is all that matters!

More Personal Experiences—Bath Time:

- First turn on the heater to make the room warm and comfortable,
- Protect carpet (if you have one),
- Turn on the water to warm up. Check the temperature for prevention of possible problems and to prevent complaints,
- Guide *mi mamacita* into the bathroom. (I said, we need to get ready to go bye-bye or tell her a therapeutic white lie,)
- I show *mi mamacita* the following: 6–8 towels, 2–4 washcloths and her clothes,
- Guide *mi mamacita* into the shower chair, and help her remove her clothes. All this time, I am singing a religious song or talking and I do not give her a chance to talk,
- Guide her into the shower and as I am singing and praying, I bathe her very rapidly. (I have found that singing religious songs are soothing to her as well as me.)
- Most of the time, I too got into the shower if I had difficulty reaching all of her body.
- Be prepared to get wet too! OOOH, the water was nice!

What a joy it is when the bath is completed! Alleluia! I always compliment *mi mamacita*. I gave her a hug and told her she smelled nice and clean. She acknowledged the compliment by smiling and saying, *"Gracias"* ("Thank you"). Of course, I have to admit this is worth a million dollars or more and guess what, I now have a clean *mamacita* to show off to the world! I never realized giving a bath to my *mamacita* was going to be such an ordeal until this first bath. A simple bath has turned out to be the ultimate ordeal. *Caramba!* (Wow!) *Gracias a Dios* (Thank-you God).

11

Activities
(*Actividades*)

After two days of living full time with *mi mamacita* on a 24/7 basis, I concluded that I could not physically nor emotionally care for *mi mamacita* alone! I needed help! This was draining me in every facet of my human being; I was totally exhausted (*¡cansada!*) to say it nicely and surprisingly, *mi mamacita* was full of energy. I immediately learned the responsibility of life in the fast lane. I learned it entailed not only a daily routine but also needed an entertainment package for *mi mamacita*. It became extremely apparent to me all kinds of "hats" are needed in order to continuously keep up with *mi mamacita*. Furthermore, interestingly enough, my nursing experiences and my experience as a mother quickly flashed into my mind like a speeding bullet or a jolt of lighting, but I was not satisfied. Whew! Of course, I will acknowledge I do not know everything but I continued to learn every day from *mi mamacita*. Amen I say to that!

I decided to call the local Alzheimer's Association again for further assistance.[1] We spoke about their assistance program and they offered Adult Day Care and At-Home Caregiver relief program as options. I knew *mi mamacita* had prior approval for the At-Home Caregiver relief program and now, Adult Day Care was being offered as my option. Day care, I thought, hmm . . . now, that is an option; after all, why not? In the meantime of waiting for my ultimate decision, I entertained *mi mamacita* the best that I could. I knew through my research that people with Alzheimer's are impatient and bored easily. I also learned that games had to be easy to play and at the same time stimulating.[4, 12] I decided to play some games that we could do together and some for her to do alone. For example: Bingo, Alphabet Cards, Number Cards, Color Books with big pictures. (I will explain more in depth later on at the end of this chapter.) After playing with *mi mamacita* for two days, I definitely could see the benefits of Adult Day Care. I must confess, I had previously felt a lady would come over to my house would be the right decision but I was most impressed seeing *mi mamacita* play and that changed my mind very fast. It was really lovely seeing her play, she was so cute. She loved the attention of doing things together. This ultimately made my decision! The very next day, I called the Coordinator at the Alzheimer's Association and told them of my decision to send *mamacita* to day care. Hurrah! I was so elated *Mamacita* was approved for three full days of day care. Hurrah! *Mi mamacita* is going to day care, I thought. Please note this was a brand new concept for me as well as for *mi mamacita*. I was most excited for us both! In my phone conversation, I was given a list of names, addresses and phone numbers of Adult Day Care centers for me to call at my convenience. After a quick review, I noted a day care which was very close to my condominium and their specialty was the care of the Alzheimer's client. Boy, I hit the jackpot, I thought. This is definitely the one I am going to call. Without hesitation, I called it immediately! The day care was most encouraging and an appointment was made to visit the next day.

Bright and early the next day, after our morning routine, I told *mi mamacita* we were going for a ride and we excitedly visited the Day Care. During our visit, we were both given a tour and I was not surprised *mi mamacita* was glued to me literally. I wondered if she sensed something "fun" about the day care? I did not tell her anything but saw the clients playing games too. Interestingly, neither she nor I said a word to each other.

After the tour, I was asked to fill out some paperwork, which I delightfully did. Then the big shock came, are you ready for this? I was told that there was a waiting list of about two to three months. You should have seen my mouth drop! Two months! WOW! I was shocked, disappointed and overwhelmed! I thought to myself, how am I going to survive doing 24/7 duty of *mi mamacita* for two MORE months? Wow, what a wait! What patience! I calmed myself down after praying quietly and rapidly to myself. Oh well, things could be a lot worse, I thought! *Mi mamacita* and I just smiled at each other. I thanked the ladies and said good-bye. I grabbed *mamacita*'s hand and we walked together like little kids going to the car, smiling the whole way.

I decided to entertain *mi mamacita* by driving around the freeway for a long drive while I pondered my next move of my survival and to calm myself down. We both listened to *mamacita*'s favorite Mexican music as she sang along. My plan did not take me long to consider; it was like the flash of a light bulb turned on and I immediately felt energized! I decided to plan an activities/entertainment program. What else could I do! Take a vacation? Go the Beach?

Please individualize your plan of care! These activities were established for *mi mamacita* only!

They are not intended as a reference but as personal experiences. If they are to be used, they must be modified for the individual person.

Activities/Entertainment Program

Car Rides: Ironically, I quickly found out *mi mamacita* loved to go out of the house on drives; anywhere, but out of the house. One day, I had to go on an errand and as I was driving, I noticed that she was smiling constantly and singing. When we returned to my house, she said, "Why are we here?" I asked her if she liked to go riding and she said, "Yes, I like the car." I also noticed when we stayed indoors, she would get anxious and frequently ask, "When are we going in the car?" This was the deciding factor in establishing car rides as an entertainment activity. I really was shocked and surprised at this new idea of car rides because when she lived alone, she would not want to go anywhere. Her home was her comfort and safe zone. *Mi mamacita* has changed, and I must adjust to her changes. (Please be aware that some people with Alzheimer's may be different because of their individual personalities. Therefore, these activities may not work!)

Before our driving adventure and the daily routines accomplished, here are a few things that I had to consider:

- Plan the trip in advance. Make sure there's enough gasoline in the car,
- Make sure that the car is in good working condition (including good tires),
- Individualize the trip,

- Do not be in a hurry, be patient and flexible,
- Take your favorite CD,
- Be prepared for any medical condition, arthritis, diabetes, etc.
- Be aware of the time of day,
- Be aware of traffic conditions, and of detour roads,
- Be aware of weather changes,
- Be aware of mood changes,
- Take snacks and money,
- Be prepared for any emergency as best as possible and have a backup plan.

I would love to share with you one of the car trips that we took. As I mentioned earlier, every trip must be individualized. Well here is an example. I guided *mamacita* to the car and applied her seat belt. I walked to the driver's side and applied my seat belts and I locked the door. As I drove down the road, I noticed she had removed her seat belt. I immediately asked her why she had removed her seat belt and she said, "It is too tight, I feel like a stuffed pig" (*"Esta cosa estar muy apretado, me siento como un marano"*). I quickly moved the car to the side of the road and parked it. I told her, "I too feel like a stuffed pig, but it is the law, we must wear our seat belts." To my surprise, she re-applied her seat belt and did keep it on for five minutes and I drove on. About two minutes later, I noted that she kept pulling on the belt and complaining and removing it. No matter what I told her, she was not satisfied and kept repeating this procedure. *Oh, mother*, I thought! I tried to distract her by singing, pointing to billboards, whatever, without success. Sometimes, distraction worked and most of the time, it did not. With frustration in my mind, this was not a good drive, but I was trying. I was determined to figure out a way of keeping on her seat belt and I prayed to myself. Finally, she kept the seat belt on for a short moment! Thank you Lord!

As we were cruising down the freeway I noticed *mi mamacita* was reading all the billboards and signs on the road. How cute, I thought. This reminded me of the days when my very own children were learning how to read and they too read the signs. My, my, I thought, how small our world is. One time, she even caught me look at her and we both smiled at each other. I also remembered my husband's suggestion of *mi mamacita*'s favorite Mexican songs CD which we played. To my surprise, she smiled and sang some of her favorite songs in Spanish. What a wonderful surprise, I thought! *Mi mamacita* singing and the seat belt is ON! We are both happy now! Thanks be to God (*Gracias a Dios*). I learned from that day forward, she loved to sing, which is a good distraction for her keeping her seat belt on. Presently, upon us getting in the car, the first thing I do is put on the Spanish CD. Miracles never cease!

Indoor Activities

Here are some activities as suggestions:

- Playing games like bingo,
- ABC's,
- Reading large picture books,
- Listening to Mexican music on the radio,
- Gardening (watering the plants),
- Small chores, like sweeping, washing dishes, folding clothes,
- Looking at family pictures,
- Watching *Novellas* (Mexican soap-operas),

- Exercise games,
- Sing-a-longs,
- Coloring (see page 114):
- Dancing: (you might even want to dance together),
- Writing: It is my practice of correspondence with the family members that wrote, or just writing down *mamacita*'s thoughts. (See pages 115 and 116.)
- Chores: One day, I recognized *mi mamacita* loved to feel wanted and needed by helping with chores. As a result, on a daily basis, I gave her the broom and asked her to help me sweep the kitchen. The next day, I asked her to sweep the bedrooms. The third day, I asked her to sweep the patio. This routine was repeated weekly. I also asked her to help me fold the clothes after they came out of the dryer. Interestingly, sometimes I repeated these same routines of folding the clothes even though they were already dry. She did not mind nor know the difference. I also reminded her to make her bed every day. She did not mind doing these chores. She smiled all the time.
- Gardening: We have a very small garden but big enough for the two of us. One day, my sister Liza visited; she brought plants because we had none. It was most beautiful and remarkable how many different plants and flowers she brought us. I just have to brag what a wonderful sister she is. She loves her *mamacita* and is extremely helpful with everything. Liza would do anything for our *mamacita* and me. She even brought us this rare Hawaiian plant which is her favorite. Amazingly, that plant has grown very fast. Each time I looked at it, I thought of Liza and of how this plant is do-

ing a Luau or something. I think this is the closest to Hawaii that we all will be going to, oh well! Thanks to *mi mamacita*'s watering skills and sunshine, this plant is growing beautifully.

• Here is our daily garden routine: *Mi mamacita* and I go out to the patio to check the soil of the plants for dryness, if they need water, I went back into the house and got the water jug and we took turns watering the plants. It is that simple! Mission accomplished!

Of course, I am proud to say, *mi mamacita* had a garden at her (other) house and *mi mamacita* had a very large yard. Her garden consisted of a few plants and many large pecan trees, which gave *mi mamacita* many pecans. I have to brag about *mi mamacita* and her pecan trees. She has quite a large, loving heart and gave all of the children who visited her many, many, many pecans. But when her mind deteriorated, we all noticed that she saved pecans everywhere in her house! Pecans were located in the kitchen, refrigerator, bathroom, washer/dryer and all the cabinets. Oh, yea, everywhere! Of course, she forgot where she saved them. She saved them so well, we even sometimes could not find them ourselves. Chuckle! Some of us played treasure hunts for the fun of it and sometimes we found them, and sometimes we did not. It was cute! Besides pecan trees in the front yard, there was this very large tree which had some fruit that we could not identify. I am embarrassed to say, until recently, my younger brother, Tony, told me that the tree had large rounded yellow fruit which tasted like grapefruit. Wow! Grapefruit! How funny, we did not know that! All those years of not knowing what kind of tree it was, we finally discovered its fruit. Life is not dull at our house!

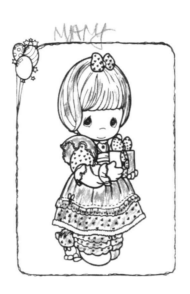

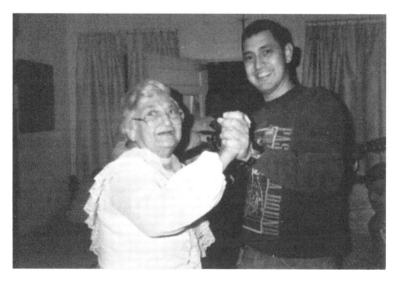

Mi Mamacita and her younger son, Tony

Antony I miss you very much
Please come home as soon as you come home
Antony I love you very much, don't
forget to call all of us at home.
Anthony we love you very much,
we want to see you soon?

Terry we love you very much,
Lots of love mom

Hilton

Mary Schultz
praying to see you soon
love mother, Mary K. Schultz

115

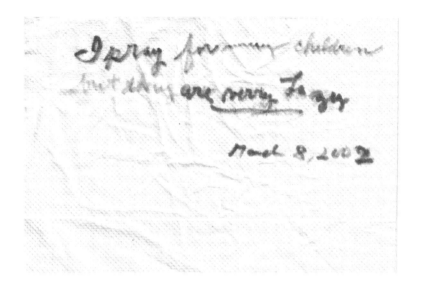

I pray for my children
but they are very lazy

March 8, 2002

- Exercise (*Ejercisio*): Yes, of course, exercise (*ejercisio*) is very important for everyone, which included *mi mamacita*. I tried to incorporate some form of exercise for her every day as well as myself, her caregiver. When she was at her old home, she walked around her yard. She also picked pecans, chased her dog and cats, swept the patio and the sidewalks. She watered her grass, plants and the patio. These are all forms of exercise and must be encouraged to be continued. Of course, I had to modify *mi mamacita*'s exercise program; it consisted of daily house exercises, household chores, garden chores and walks inside the secure gates of the condominium complex. I made sure she is dressed properly for the walk and the weather. In regards to the walks, I told her, "*Mamacita*, let us

116

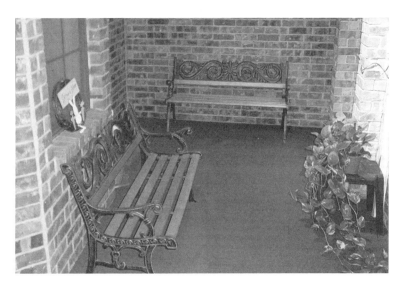

Here is a picture of our garden patio

walk and get some exercise." We held hands as we walked. These walks were short distances, because of her arthritic knees and her age. She often reminded me that "my knees hurt" (*me duele las roridas*) and we stopped for a few seconds and took a break. I reassured her of the importance of walking and we both smiled. I could tell by her smile and her comments that she enjoyed walking. One day, she exclaimed, I like to walk ("*me gustar andar.*") This made me feel good. There are some thank-you's in this type of job, let me reassure you, not too many, but take them when they come. Thanks be to God (*Gracias a Dios*).

- A Trip to the Zoo: If you decide to take this trip, I strongly suggest you take an extra person to help you. This particular day, was one of those beautiful Texas days in April. Not too hot, yet! It occurred in the spring of 2002. One day, I felt and saw the beautiful sunshine shining through my window. Please close your eyes and imagine and feel the sun rays piercing through the window! Hm . . . it sure feels good, doesn't it? It was about 10:00 in the morning. This particular day, I decided to be adventurous. Yup, I decided to take *mi mamacita* to the zoo! After breakfast, I asked her if she remembered going to the zoo when she was a child and she said, "yes, I have been to the zoo" (*"sí, yo fué al zoo."*) Well, there it was, my decision was sealed with approval, I thought! I was very excited for both of us.

I anxiously prepared us for the trip. I ensured that we girls wore comfortable clothes, walking shoes and a hat. I checked my wallet for money for cool drinks and food. Funny thing though, I could not foresee any problem. Oh shucks, I am already telling you my story, kind of, sort of. Oops, sorry about that! We got into the car, did my routine of the CD, the seat belts and started driving on the road. Alright, on the road again, I thought happily. On the drive, *mi mamacita* kept asking me, where are we going today (*"a donde vamos hoy?"*) I could not help myself, I said, "the zoo." You too would get excited to see the gleam in her eyes as well as her big smile. Oh, what a happy day, I thought, we were going to the zoo! I felt that we were lucky girls, just me and *mi mamacita*! Within a thirty-minute drive, we arrived at the zoo's parking lot. I looked for a handicap parking spot and parked the car. I placed my special handicap decal on the front of the rear view mirror as instructed. I walked to the passenger side of the car and opened her door. She immediately asked,

"Where are we going?" I answered her, "To the zoo." She got out of the car and we walked together to the zoo gate. I paid the entrance fee and we walked to the handicap area to rent a wheelchair. She smiled and sat down in the wheelchair as I pushed *mi mamacita* around to see the animals. As I was pushing, I noticed that the sidewalks were not leveled and sometimes there were hills. Whew! I exclaimed to her, "Oh, Mother, you are heavy!" This pushing is hard! I thought! Huff and puff, I went.

Well, it was not too long into this wonderful zoo adventure, about five minutes to be exact, that *mi mamacita* said, "Take me to my house." Believe, me, I nearly choked when I heard those words. Wow! Here I am pushing this wheelchair with a 145-pound *mamacita* on it and she tells me to take her home! WOW! What happened to quality time together? She has only seen two animals and she is bored already? Wow! Of course, I was upset, but I promise, I kept my cool and smiled and tried to be a good daughter. I quickly took a deep breath, prayed for patience, strength and guidance in this situation, and I quickly looked the other way as if I did not hear her. As a distraction, I continued to push her to see the other animals. I kept saying to her, oh, look at the lion, look at the zebra, etc. Five minutes later, she said again, "Take me to my home." Well, this time I was really tired of pushing and those uphill, curvy roads and the hot sun were beginning to bear down on me. Because I was tired and hot, I stopped suddenly, turned around and said to *mi mamacita*, "Mother, I want to go home too, but I am very tired and I need to rest!" I pushed the wheelchair and stopped at a shady spot under a tree and sat down for a few minutes. As I attempted to recover, *mi mamacita* again said, "Take me to my house." This time, I ignored her but pushed her and the wheelchair toward the exit shown on the map. At the end of this walkway, I saw that we were fenced in. Oh dear Lord, I said to myself, what am I supposed to do? As I turned to look at the fence, I saw construction workers and I shouted, "Please help us, we are fenced in." To make matters worse, they said, "Lady, you are in a construction area and you have to go back." I was furious, I told them that we were <u>not</u> turning back because my mother had Alzheimer's and we had to go home! I further said that there were no construction signs at the entrance and that my mother had no patience so that they had to help us get out!! I immediately got a hold of myself and told them to please call security to help us out. Within a matter of a few minutes, three security guards arrived. They were very helpful and asked me what had happened. I explained the situation and they immediately opened the fence gate and escorted us out of this fenced area. As I wheeled *mi mamacita* out, I noted by this time, other people behind us were also fenced in and they followed us out too. I was relieved and happy to get ourselves out of there. Of course, *mi mamacita* had no idea what had happened, she just smiled! Now, that was our fun trip to the zoo! What a zoo it was! To this date, we have not spoken of this incident nor have we returned to the zoo; of course I have told my husband, my sons, my brother and sister and my friends and now everybody. I hope that other people have a better experience than I did!

- Shopping: By now, one can tell each trip is an adventure of its own. To tell you the truth, it does not bother me if we encountered difficulties, they just made me stronger. I have learned they do not slow me down and prevent me from providing quality time with *mi mamacita*. Now, this next adventure is shopping at a department store. As a known fact, most stores are very cold. This time, I was prepared and brought along a sweater due to *mamacita*'s age and tendency to get cold. As always, I did not tell her where we are going but I sensed she knew. It is a known fact, every morning *mi mamacita* smiled and asked, "Where are we going today?" I guess I have spoiled her and that is okay with me. It gives me joy that she is happy!

One day, I drove to the department store close to my house. As I always do, I looked for a handicap parking spot. If I cannot find one, I then parked as close to the entrance as possible. Like silly girls ready to go shopping, we both smiled at our arrival. I placed my hand out and she held it. We walked together to the store's wheelchair section and looked for a wheelchair and I found one and guided her to sit down. At first she hesitated and said, "I do not want to sit down." I convinced her it would be a long walk and instructed her to sit down. When she sat down, she said, "I want to go to my home." I ignored her and proceeded to push the wheelchair around the store. I remembered that on previous trips to this same store, wheeling her around kept her amused for about 15–20 minutes. But within 5 minutes, she repeated, "Take me to my home." I ignored her again. I continued to wheel her around the store hoping this would distract her. I quickly thought, this visit was different; I should have known from the start, when she refused to sit down in the wheelchair. Then she said, "I am cold." What is wrong with this *mamacita* of mine? It sounded to me like a "complaint trigger switch" had been turned on in her brain and she could not stop complaining! I tried to distract her by wheeling her to different aisles of the store. To my sur-

121

prise at the top of her lungs, she suddenly shouted to the customers around us, "My daughter will not take me home." Boy, what a shock! I was absolutely stunned *mi mamacita* had the guts to say something like that. I was so embarrassed and apologized to the customers. I explained that she had Alzheimer's and of course she heard me and she exclaimed, "I don't have Alzheimer's!" Amazingly, I quickly moved her to the fish tank for further distraction with the fish; after all, she had enjoyed this spot before. At first, she was quiet and stared at the fish, she also smiled, but I noticed that she was really staring at a worker that was helping a customer with a fish selection. Within five minutes, she bursted out and said, "Help me, help me; my daughter will not take me home!" That did it, I quickly thought! The man turned around and stared at me really ugly. I was so embarrassed! Boy, I felt like a crazy woman, but that is okay, I can adjust to whatever. I carry all kinds of hats! I apologized and said, "Please forgive my mother but she has Alzheimer's." My mother yelled again, "I don't have Alzheimer's, I want to go home!" The man very politely told me to please take my mother home. I was so embarrassed, I blushed with embarrassment. I didn't know what to do. I have never been thrown out of any store! I quickly prayed! Quickly, I wheeled her to the cash register, paid for my purchases and rapidly went to our car. *Mi mamacita* just smiled as we approached the car and acted as if nothing happened. Almost instantly, she said, "Where are we going?" My mouth just dropped! What could I say? I just smiled and said, "We are going bye-bye."

• Fast food restaurants: This is one of *mi mamacita*'s favorite trips, the restaurant. I guess this is because she loves to eat; also because she does not like to wait. *Mi mamacita* and I went to the local fast food restaurants at least twice a week. I liked to take her after day care to continue to bond. This too, reminds me of when my sons were little boys and also enjoyed going to fast food restaurants. For everyone's information, her favorite foods include cheeseburger or fish burger just like the rest of us. How cute! At the restaurants, we speak very little; after all, we both know this is where we eat. These are fun times together.

- The Grocery Store (*La Tienda*): *Mi mamacita* also likes to go to the grocery store to help me shop. I know, I have said this before, and I will probably say it several more times, these trips too have been positive ones, most of the time. I did find out though, as with the other trips, that one needs to pre-plan it. Some of these include: (1) Go by yourself the first time in order to scope the area, (2) Time of day to shop to avoid traffic, (3) Handicapped parking location, (4) Location and accessibility of wheelchairs or other mode of transportation, (5) Written grocery list, (6) Sweater.

- Soap Operas (*Tele-Novellas*): I am happy to announce there are lots more fun times together, just me and *mi mamacita*! I am delighted to admit, sitting down in front of a television and watching Soap Operas (*Novellas*) is my favorite one so far! Soap Operas, one might ask? Yes! (¡Sí!) Watching them is like reviving one of my most favorite Mexican-American traditions. *Novellas* are as entertaining as the American versions of soap operas. They bring me joy to celebrate my culture with *mi mamacita*. I am sure this particular custom is as old as my great grandparents. I remember seeing my grandmother (*mi abuelita*) watching *Novellas* as I was growing up. I am sure that some of you can remember being raised with *Novellas* too. I have to admit though, watching TV is a new one for me because I do not watch TV on a regular basis. My life with my husband is quite different; there just does not seem to be any time to sit down and watch TV. Here though, I have learned to sit down and see life quite differently. My life with *mi mamacita* has totally changed me; it has taught me to sit down, relax and enjoy her and our culture. Funny thing, I have to admit, sometimes, I cannot seem to compose myself to get away from a *Novella* because I get so emotionally involved in the story. Some have captivated me to the extent that I want to continue watching them even though *mi mamacita's* attention span has been reached and she walks away. Oh, dear *mamacita.* The TV routine starts at 6 P.M. when I announce, come on *mamacita*, it is time to watch *Novellas,* let's go baby! I grab her hand and we both walk to the bedroom. I turn the TV on and we sit down for about one hour and watch *Novellas.* Yep! Of course, as you can imagine, it is not a solid hour of sitting down together. No way!! She definitely tells me when she is bored. She says, "Take me home" and I said, "Not yet, *Mamacita,*come watch with me." At times, I desperately tried to distract her so I could finish watching the *Novella.* Sometimes, I am lucky and sometimes I am not. Lucky for me, portions of *Novellas* are repeated the very next night. I am a lucky girl! Since this is the last thing that we do together before bedtime, I tried to make this experience a pleasant thing for me and *mi mamacita*, but sometimes, I have to sacrifice giving up my *Novella*, oh well, I will catch up tomorrow, I hope!

In conclusion, watching *Novellas* and doing activities together accomplished a dual purpose, that of entertaining *mi mamacita*, and taught me to appreciate and understand a different aspect of my Hispanic language, culture and my responsibility. Living with someone with Alzheimer's is a daily learning experience with a lot of adventures which have many ups/downs and many surprises! Each day is a blessing from God! *Gracias!*

12
Training Day
(*Día de Trainier*)

I must confess how I really learned to properly care for *mi mamacita*. It was not by magic, let me assure you! Let me further assure you, it was not because I am a nurse, either. I must admit, I did **NOT** know how to take care of her just because she is *mi mamacita*. Taking care of one's own family, especially a mother, is very different. I am very happy to advertise to everyone that there are now classes to learn how to care for a loved one with Alzheimer's.

I, of course, had to learn how to care for my beloved *mamacita*. I called the National Association of Alzheimer's and was directed to their local chapter in San Antonio, Texas. They were extremely pleasant and eager to help me. They immediately sent information on the available resources and directed me to a support group. The information pack included a list of classes that I could attend to learn how to take care of a loved one with Alzheimer's. Alleluia! About time! I am sure that many caregivers can conclude: caring of a loved one is no vacation or a picnic, but is done with love and obligation.

One might further ask, how in the heck did she get the idea that she had to learn how to care for her mother, after all; is this something different? Thanks for asking.

One exhausted night, after just my first week of 24/7 care, I finally sat down and reviewed the Alzheimer's Association information packet.[1] After further review, an article caught my eye, which said, Training Day classes are offered to assist a caregiver, just call for an appointment. I thought, well, I'll be! Training Classes? School? Yes, I excitedly smiled! That is for me! I need help! I need to learn how to take care of *mi mamacita* while I am waiting for the Day Care to accept her. I need more help, now and fast (*¡pronto!*) I also thought, am I really going back to school? Me, a daughter and a nurse? How cute! I never dreamed I needed to learn how to take care of *mi mamacita*. WOW! I guess one is never too old to learn. Amazing, we learn something new every day! Amazing! Without further delay, I swallowed my pride because I have no time to think about pride. I have to think about survival and how to care for *mi mamacita*. I quickly got excited and decided to call for an appointment the immediate next morning, fast (¡pronto)!

As the morning arrived with the sun peeking through my shutters, I awoke anxiously. I felt my heart rapidly beating within my chest. I heard my breath through the voice of my *mamacita* as she said, "I am hungry." Without hesitation, and like a speeding robot, I quickly ran to the kitchen and prepared breakfast for us girls. After breakfast, as I gave *mi mamacita* a magazine for distraction, I reviewed the Alzheimer's literature again. I noted one particular line: "Grace Place provides educational and training classes in the behavioral problems associated with Alzheimer's disease. Class is held on the third Wednesday of each month. For more information or to register call the number listed."[4] As I dialed the phone number, the phone menu stated the class started Wednesday, tomorrow. I thought oh, my goodness, I hope they still have room for one more student. I felt sick to my stomach with nerves because I was so very anxious and nervous; I started to breathe fast and I could hear my heart speed rapidly. I thought, what if the classes are full? What am I going to do? I dialed the phone number again as I prayed there would be space available for me. Suddenly, a soft spoken voice was heard on the other end and she said **YES** to my request. All right, I exclaimed to myself. Hurrah! Thank you, dear Jesus! I could hardly contain myself and my emotions. Finally, I was going to get some help! And to top that, they also offered to care for *mi mamacita* during my class attendance. Alleluia, I was so excited! Now, that is a double bargain, if you ask me. But I toiled with the decision to take her or get a sitter for her. I quickly came to my decision, No! I do not think so; I decided to leave her at home with my sister-in-law because I felt I needed to concentrate in the class and not on *mi mamacita* in the next room.

As one can imagine, I could not sleep that Tuesday night with the anticipation of what to expect in class the next morning. I tossed and turned at least twenty-five times. I even counted sheep or something just to convince myself I needed to learn how to care for *mi mamacita* properly. I guess I fell asleep because before I knew it, *mi mamacita* came to my bedside and woke me up, talk about reality check! I quickly arose and told myself, now that is why I need to go to school. After our morning routine, I quickly got dressed for my class. *Mi mamacita* saw me dressed and she stared at me, so I told her that I was going to work because I knew that she would not understand if I told her the truth. She looked puzzled and kept asking, "Where are we going today?" No matter what I told her, she repeated the same words many times. I finally told her that we were having a visitor, her daughter-in-law, Diana, who was coming today. After a few minutes, that answer seemed to satisfy her and she walked away without any further questions. About an hour later, Diana arrived. Since both of us are nurses, it was our routine to use the plan of care. *Mi mamacita* listened attentively and smiled. This was the first time I left *mi mamacita* and I was not worried. After all, Diana is a mother and a nurse too. What a lucky *mamacita* she was; she now had two nurses to take care of her. After my report, I turned toward the door and said, "Good-bye, mother, I am going to work." She smiled and said, "Good-bye." I closed and locked the house door, and drove off to my class. During my drive, I wondered what I was going to learn. I could feel myself anxious but at the same time confident and open-minded of this new concept.

Excitedly, I arrived at my class at 9:00 A.M. sharp and got out of the car. Like my first day of school, I hurriedly walked to the door and rang the doorbell. I saw a woman walk to the door holding a chain of keys while she unlocked the door. While she approached and unlocked the door, she was smiling with a smile of confidence. After her greeting, she explained the day care doors were locked to prevent any wandering clients. The woman asked for my name and for my purpose. I told her I was attending the training class and she walked me to the classroom. During this walk, we passed by some clients; I saw them playing games. I was most impressed to see a structured program. They appeared happy as they were smiling. She showed me the classroom and asked me to wait. I sat down and looked around and noticed I was in a conference room and I was the only student. There were tables and chairs surrounded with book shelves. A few minutes later, a very calm-looking woman came in and introduced herself as the instructor. She was very nice and professional but not personal. At the beginning of the class, the instructor did not ask any information about me nor *mi mamacita*. She started her class as a matter of fact by explaining facts about Alzheimer's. I could tell by her voice and the method of her explanation that she was very knowledgeable. She gave me brochures and showed me audio-visual aids. She introduced me to the library and explained its policy. She asked me if there were any specific problems in my taking care of *mi mamacita*. I smiled and said, yes. We had an in-depth discussion on baths, hunger and wanting to go home. She reassured me that these were common problems and I would learn how to handle them. She gave me specific brochures to assist me. I thanked her and felt relieved and happy.

Out of curiosity, I must admit, every so often, I turned around to check if anybody else had come in during the class and no one else was present in the room, to my surprise, I was by myself. Would anyone believe that I AM THE CLASS? I FELT SPECIAL! I thought, How swell! I am the class! These people really care about my *mamacita* and me!

About two hours later, the Program Director walked in. All of a sudden the room seemed very quiet and one could almost imagine a pin drop. Her presence deserves that much respect! Just by her walk and her smile, one could tell this woman knew the material that she was going to tell me. To top it off, she had not even opened her mouth yet! When our eyes made contact, she introduced herself to me, the class! Her mannerisms immediately impressed me! I would like to refer to the expression, first impressions are the best and lasting ones; well, this woman fitted that one like a glove! We sat down and she said, "How is your mom?" What a question to start our first meeting. I felt content that she asked me about *mi mamacita.* It was like our friendship was sealed! We continued our class and talked a lot! She emphasized the importance of a caregiver acquiring this special education, and the importance of support of other caregivers as well as respite care. Amen, I said to that, to myself of course. She gave me a schedule of the dates of the support group. She further emphasized the importance of establishing a routine and sending our loved one to Day Care. She asked me if *mi mamacita* was already in Day Care and I said no. I informed her that *mamacita* was approved but was on the waiting list. She acknowledged the fact of the waiting list and apologized. But she reassured me the waiting period would pass soon and gave me some day care activity schedules to assist me. Our class concluded with a tour of the Day Care. When I left, I was most impressed of my training day. I felt good! Once I got into my car, I decided to review these materials to determine how I was going to practice what I had just learned.

The Day Care activity schedule included:

(a) names of games that were rotated every twenty minutes, like playing ball, bingo, cards, dominoes, (b) beauty shop days which were held weekly, (c) trips, (d) sing-a-longs, (e) exercise classes, (f) storybook reading.[4]

That same night, after *mi mamacita* was asleep, I reviewed the materials that she gave me and I sighed with a sense of relief and took a deep breath, AHHHHHHHH! I felt a peace within my heart and closed my eyes. I thanked God for my class today and asked him for continued guidance and strength!

13

My Husband Visits Us!
(¡*Nos Visita Mi Marido!*)

This chapter is like a romantic fairy tale. Yes, fairy tales are still around. How cute! I am delighted to say this because this is how I felt each weekend my husband came to visit. I am so lucky and blessed! Yes, yes, believe it! My husband flew down from Washington, D.C. to visit *mi mamacita* and me every weekend! Yup, he sure did! Now that is Love! (¡*Amor!*) His love is so strong that he wanted to be part of my new life with *mamacita*. *He is my Prince Charming! Please imagine, every weekend, this Prince Charming coming down and visiting us girls? After a whole week of stress, stress, stress, we girls welcomed him warmly and with open arms, literally! Now that is genuine love (amor)!* Ok, enough for mushiness . . . SMILE!!

Yes, of course, I gladly admit, *mi mamacita* and I looked forward to seeing my husband each weekend. Upon his arrival, we girls smiled and greeted him with kisses and hugs like some silly little girls. That was fun and most rewarding to us all! It was like a cheerful welcoming. The weekends were very different for all of us. We did special things together. We went to church, breakfast, all our meals, drives and special trips. My husband and I made weekends special for *mi mamacita* and us. That is why this is a romantic fairy tale! My husband arrived very late every Thursday and *mi mamacita* did not get the opportunity to greet him until the next morning because she was asleep. Every Friday morning, when *mamacita* woke up, I saw that she had a gleam in her beautiful brown eyes with a very big smile each time she saw my husband approach her bedroom door. When she first saw him, her face gleamed and her first words were "Who are you?" My husband answered, "I am Juan, Terry's husband." She smiled and said, "I did not know that!" She was so cute and sincere with those words. *Mi mamacita* and my husband had a special bond together. He always made her smile and laugh. I am a lucky daughter with a very understanding and loving husband. I am blessed! They had many conversations together which lasted only a few minutes but seemed like hours because they always laughed. I am happy to have observed them having a good time together. I am happy and pleased of his visits. Like I said, he is our Prince Charming!

The goal of my husband and I was to make every weekend happy, fun and rewarding for all of us, which they were.

Here are some of the activities that we accomplished:

Church (*La Iglesia*)

My husband and I decided to take *mi mamacita* to church every Sunday as per our religion. Most importantly, the decisions we faced were, which church and what day, Saturday or Sunday? Before we made our decision, we needed to check the availability of handicap ramps as well as quiet rooms. We proceeded on this expedition by concluding these answers would be determined by trial and error. Okay, here goes . . . we tried different churches and different times for a couple of weeks. After several attempts, my husband and I concluded to take *mi mamacita* to a sermon which was in Spanish and hopefully she could participate better. Alleluia! Amen! We hit the jackpot! It was beautiful to see *mi mamacita* actually pray and sing in her language; it was most impressive! I saw the smile on her face and the gleam in her eyes while she was having a good time. She looked beautiful, just like a beautiful little girl, almost like an angel. I felt real proud of her. I must admit though, that she does not always repeat this beautiful scene often and therefore we were happy when these rare moments occurred. On those moments whereby she got tired or bored with church, she said, "When is the Mass over?" I, of course, tried to reassure her and tried to explain that the sermon was almost finished and encouraged her to pray, which at that particular time, it worked.

Eating Out (*Azenar*)

As I have mentioned many times before, *mi mamacita* loves to eat, that includes going out to restaurants. Every Friday, Saturday and Sunday after church, *mi marido* (husband) took us to lunch or dinner. We drove to the Malt House, which was one of her favorite restaurants in the west side of town where my parents used to live together. I recalled many happy memories of this Mexican restaurant. It is a favorite hangout for Mexican-Americans who lived in that neighborhood. I too went there as a child and as an adult. The restaurant has *Mariachias*, a Mexican singing group, and we all enjoyed their music. This was our favorite restaurant until one day, my husband and I noticed my mother moving restlessly about the car. At the restaurant, we also noticed that she got impatient on the length of time the food was delivered to our table. She even shouted, "Where is my food? I am hungry!" I had to calm her down by distraction of looking at the other people. Oh well, It was fun while it lasted! This particular incident taught me the importance of my responsibility of flexibility and patience. Okay, give me a break, I am trying!

Driving Around in the Car/Cruising (*Travesiando*)

This may sound somewhat silly, but *mi mamacita* loved to be in the car. It really was somewhat funny because my husband and I planned our daily drives and tried to have long drives. Okay, here we go on one of our drives, everybody, get your seatbelts and sunglasses on and turn on the radio or CD (Vicente Fernandez).[14] My husband and I laughed when we reminisce we were always in the streets. Foolishly, I have to smile and say besides the usual drives to church and the restaurant, we took longer drives to several different areas. Examples are: the park, the store, around the freeway, to visit friends and family or just around the block; anywhere because she liked to be in the car. Most of our drives were successful but not all of them. Ironically, family and friend visits were not successful trips. *Mi mamacita* did not like to sit still at people's houses; it must be the motion of the drives that pacified her, I would conclude. For whatever reason, I immediately noticed as she arrived at family and friend's house, she would exclaim in a very loud voice, "Let's go, I have a headache." I tried to distract her by changing the subject but this did not work. I thought to myself, this was amazing, how she communicated her likes or dislikes. She had her own line of defense which she communicated to us easily. Sometimes, I ignored her until she insisted by repeating those words, "Let's go, I have a headache," and of course after about fifteen minutes of these repeats, we left. At first, my husband and I were embarrassed but we rapidly learned this was her way of letting us know she was bored. Very amazingly, as soon as we got in the car, her headache was gone and she smiled and sang as we drove along the freeway. WOW!

Talk about flexibility, yea, we aimed to please! I can honestly vouch that we should get a grade of A for patience and flexibility! Hurrah! Sometimes, we felt that my *mamacita* graded us, just kidding! It was most obvious that everything we did was for *mi mamacita*! Happy days are here today, oh happy days are here today! Thanks to God!

The Beach (*La Playa*)

OK, everybody, it is summertime and we must go to the beach (*la playa*). Now get your beach towel, beach ball and do not forget that sun tan lotion! I exclaim with excitement that going to the beach is the ultimate summer vacation! This time, we are going to the beach with *mi mamacita*, hurrah! HOWEVER, I do have to **PRE-WARN, DO NOT DO IT ALONE! TAKE ANOTHER PERSON TO HELP YOU OUT BESIDES THE DRIVER!**

Why drive to the beach one might wonder when it is about 150 miles away? I guess, I must admit, because of my optimism, I wanted to give back to *mi mamacita* some of the joy she gave us as children. Going to the beach (*la playa*) was part of our annual summer vacation. Those were some of the good times of my family. I dearly remember the beach, playing on the sand, fishing and sleeping on the floor of our rented beach house. Good memories! One Saturday morning, I asked my mother, do you remember when you and Dad took us children to the beach for summer vacations? She immediately smiled and said, yes!

As one can imagine, there were no second thoughts on my part when she said yes, we were definitely going to the beach. Hurrah! Like little kids, my husband, *mi mamacita* and I immediately rushed into the car. I noticed as I tried to place her seatbelt on, she burst out and said, "Where are we going today?" I told her we were going to the beach and she smiled! Now, please humor me and imagine the three of us, in the freeway, singing with Vicente Fernandez and all of us smiling. What a picture perfect moment that I will keep in my memory department. A scene of a happy family if you ask me! Oh, yea, we all looked like one big happy family! Of course, we stopped for a break, two or three breaks to be exact, but that was alright. We ate ice cream, cookies and other goodies. Two hours later, we arrived at the beach, happy and smiling. My husband and I gave a sigh of relief that the drive went very well. Like a common statement, no problem. Whew! Upon our arrival, we stopped at the local fast food restaurant because of course we were all hungry. We ordered our beach picnic lunch which consisted of hamburgers and French fries. My husband then drove us to the beach and parked the car, finally! With excitement, the three of us exclaimed how beautiful the day was and how big the waves were. We could feel the warm breeze on our faces and saw the waves crest on the beach. "Oh, what a beautiful day," I said. My mother also said, "Look at the bird on the beach." We ate our hamburgers and watched the children laughing and playing in the water. I was so excited of this happy moment that I called on the cell phone my younger brother, Tony, and sister, Liza, and shared this special moment. After eating, *mi mamacita* and I walked together along the beach. We smiled as we enjoyed the wind and sun blowing across our faces. It was a beautiful few moments of our lives together. How beautiful, I thought! All of a sudden, I looked at my watch and noticed that it was 5:00 P.M. and realized it was getting late! I told my husband we had better get back to San Antonio *pronto* (fast) because I knew that we had to get back home before dark because of the "sun-down syndrome."[1, 8] We did not want to risk *mi mamacita*'s paranoia to get worse. I do admit, that we were having such a wonderful time that I was not aware we had been gone about five hours. Hurriedly but patiently, I grabbed *mi mamacita*'s hands and we walked to the car. After she got into the car, I placed her seat belt on, locked the doors, put the Mexican CD, "Vicente Fernandez" on and my husband drove on back to the freeway and to San Antonio. Within thirty minutes, I heard a noise in the back seat which sounded like a rope being pulled. I also heard her loud voice. I turned immediately around to the back seat and noticed my mother was pulling on her seat belt, pulling on the door lock and shouting, "Take me home and take this belt off." All of a sudden, she reached her arm to my husband who was driving the car and I immediately grasped her hands and moved them away. Talk about tense moments! And, oh, my goodness . . . I quickly distracted *mi mamacita* by pointing to the outside of the window and directing her eyes to outdoor activities. As my heart raced, I counted the cows, horses, cactus, and other cars. At the same time, I instructed my husband to stop the car at the nearest gas station. I also placed my arm across my husband to prevent *mamacita* not to touch him. This distraction worked for only a few minutes. I continued to count and she firmly said, "I already did that." Wow! I was stunned! It was a big time challenge trying to distract her, let me say. We finally arrived at a gas station and we got out of the car and took a break to cool off. This break seemed to have helped a little. After fifteen minutes, we got back into the car and my husband drove again. To our surprise, *mi mamacita* continued to throw the same tantrum almost five minutes later. I continued to try to distract her and protect us. Oh, goodness gracious, it was awful and scary. In between these nerve-wracking episodes, I prayed and sang to try to distract *mi mamacita*. Two hours later, finally, we arrived home, safely! Thanks be to God! What a trip, my husband and I thought! It was a horrible drive back! It was like a nightmare that we could not stop. I concluded that, I guess, *mi mamacita* was tired and did not know how to express herself any other way. From that date forward, we decided to better plan the time element of our trips. We also concluded that we learn something every day. We said to ourselves that we must recognize the signals *mi mamacita* shows us and we have to know how to respond to them; after all, she is totally dependent on us.

In conclusion, we must continue to pray to make the right decisions.

14
Taking Care of Oneself—
Respite Care
(*Cuidandose*)

What is a caregiver one might ask? A caregiver is a very special person who works 24/7 or 24 hours a day, 7 days a week, 365 days a year to be more specific! Hello there, can anybody do this type of job and not get tired? How about payment? No, I do not think so! Does this person deserve some time off? What about vacation? Oh yea! We who are caregivers are not robots or super humans, wish we were though! What is Respite Care? Are you tired? Well, if you are tired, do you want Respite Care? Funny thing, I too, had to learn what Respite Care means because it is not an everyday word, especially in my Hispanic/Latina vocabulary or culture. Here we go learning again. . . . Respite Care means care for the caregiver.[1, 4, 5, 6, 8, 10] How about that! Well, how interesting the concept of taking time off for oneself; this thing of Respite Care, now that sounds like I, as many of my people have been missing out on. Now, this is too bad because we all must learn the importance of taking care of ourself.

In my culture, one does not think of caring for oneself **FIRST**![7] Family comes **FIRST,** no matter what! That is our life! Does anyone remember one's *mamacita* taking a

day off from caring for you when you were a child? Hmmm
. . . I don't think so. Respite Care, now that sounds interesting. My, my, how life has changed! Through my research, it reinforced the fact, a person is a better
caregiver when one cares for oneself **FIRST**! [1, 4, 6, 7, 8]
Hmm, I thought, that is absolutely correct! For a few minutes, I thought, wait a minute, as if a light bulb turned on.
As educated Hispanics, we must try to change that old
theory of family comes **first**. [7]

I must say, this is an interesting concept because it
really makes sense. Hmm . . . this first puzzled me because taking care of oneself first was not the way I was
raised. I was raised like most Hispanic families; that family came first, no matter what! I am sure that some readers can remember taking care of a loved one even though
one was sick too. Never, ever did that person take time
off! I know for a fact, and I am sure not all *mamacitas* ever
took personal leave when children were born or sick.
There was no such thought of that! Amazing how some
things have changed! Sadly, at the same time, I think
that some of my Hispanic people will not change entirely
and that is OK too, whatever works for each family.

Now, please close your eyes and try to think back to
when you were a child. Did your parents take some time
off? Most probably not! If yes, great! If not, that is like my
culture. Now, close your eyes again and pretend you are a
parent. Have you gone out with your husband or your
friends? If you did go out, it was fun, wasn't it? Yes, of
course, it was fun! And you were re-energized to face the
children and the world, right? When you returned, were
the children OKAY? Of course they were, right? Of
course, they survived and so did you! Amazing, isn't it,
and such a simple concept! We just have to convince the

rest of the world how simple and important respite care is. It is almost common sense. SMILE!

Several years ago, when I was a mother with young children at home, I too remember taking time off with my husband and my friends. Let me tell you the secret which has worked for me. Very early on in our marriage, my husband told me the importance of nourishing our marriage by going out on dates. I thought, what is he talking about? We are married! We don't need dates anymore. "What are you talking about?" I asked him. "I am too busy with the children, work and besides, I am tired. Are you crazy or something? Please open your eyes!" Afterwards, one night, my husband sat me down and told me our children were here for a short length of time under our wings and one day grow up and move away to college, get married and we would be alone as husband and wife. Question, would we know each other if we never had time for each other? Nope! Wow, what a question? Now, I thought, this is a very loaded question! He further stressed we, Mom and Dad, husband and wife, must have the foundation and responsibility for them and for ourselves. We must not forget ourselves as husband and wife. If we do not nourish our marriage, we would not know each other! Now, how about that Hispanic thinking! I, at first, did not understand him but I believed him and it has worked, I am proud to say! I am a lucky wife, my husband made it a practice for us to go out to dinner once a week and I have thanked him many, many times since then. We also took personal and family vacations every year. Oh, yea, that was a lot of fun too. On personal vacations, we explained to our children the purpose, which was to make us better parents. Did it work? Of course it did! The children believed us and they loved staying with friends and relatives. They too had a vacation from their parents, hurrah!

I honestly feel our family bonds grew stronger as a result of these same values. Now that is a sample of Respite Care which can be followed into different situations.

Yes, time off, or Respite Care, as it is called today, makes a lot of sense for the caregiver. One has to recognize and accept the fact that rest is needed and really make the effort to locate a sitter. I strongly feel this is a frame of mind thing. Just remember that your loved one depends on you for everything, 24/7 of it! That is it! Furthermore, the quantity of time off depends on several factors as well as the individual caregiver. These factors include, of course, a qualified sitter, the amount of time needed and the cost. There are different ways to take some time off, for example, for the hour, a few hours, for the night, a weekend or a week. Whatever works for the individual caregiver. Just do it! Swallow your pride; you are as important as your loved one that needs you! Just do it! You will be glad that you did, I did!

Before I was scheduled for some Respite Care, I learned some techniques of coping. As I read the Day Care Newsletter,[4] I read a notice about a caregiver study that I could join to learn these techniques. I immediately called and signed up for the study by the University of Texas Health Science School entitled: "Stress-Busting Program for Caregivers." This research study consisted of relaxation therapy (techniques or methods to help learn how to relax and cope with stress) and was provided to caregivers for individuals with Alzheimer's Disease.[6] Now, I smile and say thanks to the study program. I strongly believe that God (*Dios*) sent me an angel to take care of me and for me to take care of my mother. Thank you! (¡*Muchas Gracias!*)

Upon my first visit as well as weekly visits, I was attached to electrodes pads which measured my breathing

143

as well as heartbeat as I answered stress test questions. I was glad I was not facing a mirror because I felt like an astronaut attached to all kinds of wires, no offense of course is implied. I felt very different and weird with all these wires attached to me. At the beginning and end of each session they also drew blood from my arm, which was part of the procedure. Boy, those test questions, some of them were mind-boggling like reading and saying numbers backwards; wow, it was amazing how data was obtained. Overall, I am proud to say, I learned some stress-relief techniques such as listening to relaxation tapes, mental imaging, exercise and deep breathing techniques.[6]

Another thing I did was join a support group, walked nightly and wrote this book. Other forms of relaxation techniques include Yoga, karate, bird watching, gardening, shopping, movies, and bio-feedback.[6] There are many other ways to relax; one just has to learn what works best and do it! Enjoy yourself! Come on now! Here are some more techniques I learned from the caregivers study:

Ten Tips for Family Caregivers:

Caregiver is a job and respite is your earned right. Reward yourself.

- Watch out for signs of depression and do not delay in getting professional help,
- Accept the offer when someone volunteers to care for your loved one,
- Educate yourself,
- Be open to technologies and ideas,
- Trust your instincts,

- When grieving comes, dream your dreams,
- Stand up for your rights, you are not alone,
- Seek support,
- Be good to your back and the rest of your body.[5]

It is now time for me to share how I practiced Respite Care. Within the first two weeks of my caring for my *mamacita*, yes, I was tired and exhausted! Yes, me, her daughter, the nurse, was tired! I am blessed and proud to say that Diana, my sister-in-law, volunteered to help me out. Hurrah! One day, my younger brother, Tony, called and told me that his wife, Diana, was in the process of arranging her schedule to be able to provide care for *mamacita* one day every week. I thought to myself, now, that is wonderful! I jumped with joy as I heard these words because I do have to brag of course. Diana is also a Nurse; she understands about stuff like this. I further thought what a lucky *mamacita*. She now has two nurses taking care of her. Nurse Diana to the rescue, I thought! What a beautiful thing! As I anxiously waited for next Tuesday, it could not have come sooner. Frequently, I remember pacing the hallways, and looking at the calendar and at the clock. Like a silly girl, I waited and waited for the days to pass until Tuesday would arrive because I guess I must have been anxious and really looking for some personal time off. Finally, Tuesday arrived! Whew! It was definitely a beautiful day; the sun with its beautiful rays was shining brightly through the shutters and *mamacita* and I could not contain ourselves, we both smiled continuously like children. Not a word of Diana coming today was spoken by me because I did not know how *mi mamacita* was going to react. As I looked at the clock on the wall again, it definitely said 9 A.M. but I could not trust my excitement and of course doubted myself; I had to do a double take to ensure that it definitely said 9 A.M. I peeked through my window shutters to catch a glimpse of Diana driving up to our driveway as the sound of the engine roared. Diana parked her car and I could hear my heart go pitter patter in a rapid pattern as she knocked on the door. Immediately and without reservation, I opened the door with my mighty strength that it surprised us both that we chuckled and smiled. Upon my *mamacita* seeing Diana, *mamacita* said, "Who is she?" Diana smiled and said she was Anthony's wife, and to our welcome surprise, *mamacita* smiled and said, "I didn't know that!" WHEW! I was most surprised and pleased; their bond was immediately sealed. Hurrah! I told *mamacita* that I was going to work (not really—white lie, remember?), but before one could count to three, I flew out the door like a speeding bullet without looking back. As a nurse, I had pre-written the plan of care and gave an oral report on *mamacita*'s care of course. As the morning passed, of course, I called to check on *mi mamacita*, just like a mother hen caring for her chicks. After that reassuring call, I was elated to have some time to myself. It felt exhilarating and invigorating if I do say so myself! On my first Respite Care, I went to the grocery store and ran errands. As weeks passed, I thought to myself (as my light bulb turned on), wait a minute, I think this is my personal time off, I should spend it for myself. After that inspiring moment, each Tuesday thereafter, I went shopping and lunch with my girl friends. Hurrah! It was most rewarding and refreshing to have my personal time off. At 3 P.M. I returned home. I asked Diana how the day went and she gave me an oral report. During our report, I asked her what kind of activities they accomplished and she told me she interviewed *mi mamacita* on her children and wrote them down, somewhat like historical letters. I have enclosed one of these for your reading pleasure: (see pages 148 and 149)

These are just a few examples of Respite Care. I am sure that one can do whatever one can dream to accomplish the goals of rest and relaxation. Good luck, enjoy and get some Respite Care!

My name is
Mary R. Schultz

My mother's name
is Manuela Montez

My Father's Name is
Jose Montez

I have a lot of
brothers and sisters

My Husband and I used
to love to go dancing.
It was at Laredo and
Guadalupe. We used
to go there very often.
We would Walk there
and back home until
we got very tired.
We would go with my
Sisters and brothers
to dance there.
My oldest daughters
would take care of
the children. I liked
all of the dances with Ray.

15
My Sister, Liza, Visits Us!
(¡Mi Hermanita, Liza, Nos Visita!)

My sister, Liza, visited fairly often. I am so very blessed to have a sister like Liza. She too had a special bond with our mother. When she visited, we enjoyed our *mamacita* together. There was no better joy or comparison between two sisters taking care of our elderly *mamacita*. Like the saying goes, "two is better than one;" that was good for us too. We took turns with the actual responsibility of our mother because she was a handful, or shall I say, two handfuls! I think our *mamacita* was aware we were her daughters, I hope that she was! We will never know this but we both felt that she was. Together, we have seen our *mamacita* the happiest we have ever seen her. It was fun! We are blessed and lucky daughters, Liza and I. We ate together at the fast food restaurants, we went shopping together; we even took turns bathing our *mamacita*, as well as putting her to bed at night. Each of Liza's visits were always adventurous and wonderful ones. She is multi-talented and loves to sew and when she came, she brought her sewing machine. She sewed some curtains and a bedspread for one of my empty bedrooms and she made our *mamacita* some clothes too. Liza is something else! I am a lucky sister!

On many of those visits, after our mother was asleep,

Liza and I stayed up most of the night talking. Just like girls, talking, talking, talking! It was fun! Sometimes, we watched movies on the television or VCR. We are the best of sisters and this sealed our bond!

One other day, my little sister was so mischievous that she called our *mamacita* on her cell phone because our *mamacita* said, "I am lonely, nobody calls me." Liza and I looked at each other and said, "We are right here!" So, guess what, to my amazement, Liza called our *mamacita* on the cell phone from another room. I was so embarrassed, but our poor *mamacita* did not know the difference. But you should have seen our *mamacita*'s eyes gleam; she was most excited to talk to my sister. I heard them visiting and laughing loudly. Later, privately, Liza and I laughed but felt happy that she provided some laughter to our *mamacita*. I am happy to say, each time that Liza came, we three had a lot of fun!

On another Liza visit, she brought her three daughters, Lisa, Valerie and Sarah, because as a mother herself, Liza felt the importance for them to see their grandmother. She wanted them to see the importance of family and culture firsthand. As a saying goes, we can talk to our children about this, and it goes in one ear and out the other; but of course, it is better for them to see it with their own eyes. It is that special! I totally agree with my sister, Liza. I am proud that she took this opportunity to share our family and culture with her daughters.

Speaking about special, I have to share with you another very special incident. One other day, we both decided to take a nap. To be quite honest, we were both quite exhausted! It just kind of happened! Our *mamacita* had overwhelmed us at the same time with her beautiful, constant attention. We had been taking care of our *mamacita* for awhile, when suddenly, we each laid down for a nap in separate rooms without informing each other. What a crazy thing one might say! Guess what? Amazing as it sounds, it is the honest truth! We both had the same idea without consulting each other! Amazing, it must be mental telepathy or family craziness. I remember vividly, in the background of my mind, I heard our *mamacita* go from room to room and saying, "Hello, is anybody here?" "Hello!" You can be reassured, neither Liza nor I really took a deep nap because in between my mother pacing and calling out, how could we! To this date, we both chuckle with tears in our eyes about this silly incident! Can you imagine that? *Mamacita* has two daughters and both were asleep on the job! Wow, what a crazy thing we did, my mother would say; if she had a normal brain. Oh, my Lord!

On another silly visit, Liza was alone with our *mamacita* and Liza decided for the two of them to watch television. Within a short time period, Liza closed her eyes to rest for a few seconds. Oh, yea! Sleep? Nap? Right! No way, José, as our *mamacita* would say. Liza then heard *mamacita* asking for permission to lock the door because she was afraid. Liza nodded her head in the position of YES! After a few minutes, Liza opened her eyes and to her total amazement, *mamacita* barricaded the door with a movable bedside table with a chair on top of it. Liza was stunned! How could this be, our beloved *mamacita*, with Alzheimer's and arthritis, how did she do this? Our beloved *mamacita* who always complained, how did she do this? Yep, that is our *mamacita*! Liza said she dropped her mouth in amazement and stared at our *mamacita*. Liza was so shocked that she left this barricade untouched for me and *mi hermanito*, Tony, could see it. It was one of those things; believe it or not, you must see it to believe it! One thing I would love to know is, can anybody answer the question as to how our *mamacita* did this? How could she do it? Magic, I have concluded! No, I really believe people with Alzheimer's really do have super powers, I really believe! I have seen it with my very own brown eyes. Wow!

Since this day forward, I took extra care and watched *mi mamacita*, especially at night because strangely, it seems she has special powers at night too. I had already seen strange things around my house and I have personally seen *mi mamacita* wander in her bedroom looking and staring at things. I have seen her look into her cabinet drawers and look at her clothes and papers. She rolls the toilet paper into balls and hides them everywhere. She looks out at the window and walks to the doors many, many times and checks them (including the closet) and ensures that they are locked at least 20–50 times. If I questioned *mamacita*, she said, "Are the doors locked?" I answered, yes. I would hug her and say, "*Mamacita*, go to sleep." She would go back to her bed and fall asleep almost immediately. She did this scenario six–ten times every night.

One night, my husband told me that he was afraid that I would end up with a bump on my head or some other accident and advised me to sleep in the adjacent room. Let me further explain why my husband was afraid for my safety. Because *mi mamacita* was very religious all of her life and she has a lot of large ceramic statues and pictures decorating her bedroom. Strangely, I have to admit, yes, I have seen them rearranged in the same room and not by me! I guess she must have done this while I was asleep. Please note as a personal experience, protect yourself as well as your loved one. They do not know what they are doing!

16

Mamasitting
(*Cuidando a Mamacita*)

I advertise to everyone about a new job that is available for certain qualified people, it is called Mamasitting . . . which is another form of Respite Care. Is there anyone out there interested? Oh, come on now, it is not that bad. It is an experience of your life that you will never forget and would make you appreciate life a little differently, if I might add. Hurrah! Time for Terry to go out of town, I must exclaim! I brag and say that I have another guardian angel and she is my younger sister, Liza. Yes, I am a lucky girl! Whenever I asked her to care for our *mamacita*, she gladly said, YES because I traveled about 1–2 weeks every other month with my husband on his work trips and I was concerned this would be eliminated. Believe me; I looked forward to the trips! Hurrah! Terry goes out of town!

As a background, Liza had cared for our *mamacita* at her Houston home several times before I moved down to San Antonio. But this is the first time in San Antonio. In addition, I delightedly add, Liza always took care of our *mamacita* each time I went out of town. There is no other better-qualified person to care for our *mamacita* than Liza, I confirmed. Liza is a mother herself of two young beautiful daughters. She has raised seven children, along with cats, dogs, birds, gerbils, you name it, and she has raised them all. Whew!

Okay, enough bragging and of me being silly. One particular beautiful Saturday in the late afternoon in March; Liza arrived in San Antonio for two weeks. She arrived with a smile in her face as our *mamacita* smiled too. She arrived in her white Suburban. Okay, I need to explain what a Suburban is to those of you who do not know. A Suburban is the official car of Texas (not officially, of course). Ha! Ha! We Texans think so, anyway! This vehicle is really BIG. One can pack everything in it, including a kitchen sink, just about. Ha! Ha! Almost everyone in Texas has a Suburban. Anyway, it is so big! One has to ask, really how big is it? It is sooooooo big that Liza even brought her sewing machine. A sewing machine? I thought, does she think she is going to sew? Boy, this girl is in for surprise, or am I in for surprise? Let me explain a little more; Liza is also a seamstress so she brought her sewing machine. Can our *mamacita* surprise us both? We shall see.

Liza's, time with *mi mamacita*, from what I can conclude, was like "motherly bonding" for them. Below, I asked Liza to write some thoughts of her caring for our *mamacita*. Here they are: "We were *solitas* (alone), with no distractions from kids and all the familiar things that I am used to. Neither one of us felt like we were at HOME. She regularly asked me to take her HOME. She did not just ask, sometimes she would beg. I quickly learned the art of distraction, a skill I learned from raising children. I often asked her if she could wait five minutes before I would take her home. She was always agreeable. Those five minutes often turned into '*todo el dia!*' (the whole day!) Sadly, her HOME no longer exists and there is no way to get this across to her. *Pobecita mamacita* (Poor mother). I had to learn how to take care of MOM and continue to be MOM with my daughters. I had left them under the dad's care; after all, they are eleven and fourteen and can care for themselves. But, as a mother, I had to keep in touch with my girls. I decided to buy us all cell phones. I was at first hesitant due to budget restraints, but it is worth it I have found. I also drove to Houston, which is four hours away, but MOM did not seem to mind. After all, she loves drives. She did not sense what I was doing. Just driving down the freeway, seeing my girls, and turning BACK around to San Antonio. All in the same day! I figured, what the heck, MOM has nothing better to do with her time, so we drove to Houston a few times and back the same day."

How crazy was that? Besides these crazy drives, Liza told me they spent their two weeks together playing games, going to the department stores, and driving around the San Antonio freeways many, many times. Ironically, I said to myself, these are the same things I did with our *mamacita*, how funny, I thought. When I returned, *mamacita* smiled as she always does and did not notice that I was gone. I was happy that our *mamacita* had a wonderful time with her daughter, Liza, too.

As time passed, well, ready or not, it is another time for *mamacita* to go traveling out of town. It is time for Terry to go out of town, again! Oh, yea! This time, my *mamacita* travels to Houston, Texas. Yea! *Mamacita* goes to Houston! On this trip, Liza could not come down to San Antonio and as a result, we silly sisters had to think and coordinate the logistics of this trip. Some of the questions we had thought of: how does *mamacita* go to Houston? Fly or per car? Does Liza pick her up or do I drop her off? Will she be able to tolerate the drive or the airplane? How will she tolerate being out of her home environment and her routine for two or three weeks? It was very interesting planning *mamacita*'s trip. Interestingly, it was the same as planning a vacation or for babysitting but this was for *mamacita*. After consultation with Liza, we both decided for her to come down to San Antonio and pick up our *mamacita*!

There was this particular Saturday afternoon in May, as the sunshine beat hard in South Texas and Liza drove down to San Antonio. Yes, she came in her white Suburban. Again, I will say, really how big is it? It is sooooooo big that we packed all of *mamacita*'s belongings including the potty-chair. Now, that was a sight to see! It was funny packing this Suburban, and one could think we were all crazy; I guess we were, come to think of it! We chuckled and reminisced about our vacation travels in a car with the whole family when we were children. As we packed, we laughed and laughed of all the stuff that was needed. Talk about packing, we concluded everything was needed to be packed.

- Potty chair
- Shower chair
- Clothes
- Suitcase
- Toiletries
- Medicines

Finally, we were packed and it was time to drive to Houston. Finally! Whew! As I stood by the fence, I waved good-bye to *mi mamacita* and Liza. *Mamacita* smiled and waved good-bye, too. I saw Liza assist our *mamacita* to the designated passenger front seat and put on the seat belt. Funny, though, *mamacita* did not know where she was going and it did not matter. *Mamacita* knew she was going bye-bye and that is all that mattered. My concern though, it was late and night time and the drive was four hours long. Liza and I kissed thank-you and good-bye as she drove off for a <u>very</u> long drive in the moonlit sky.

Anxiously and nervously, I waited and waited to hear of their status. Within thirty minutes of being on the road, I could not help myself and I called Liza. One can probably say I was apprehensive but no, I was just concerned and I wanted to talk to *mi hermanita*. Quickly, I dialed her cell phone and I asked her about *mamacita* and her toleration, thank goodness for cell phones! Liza told me that she was OK so far. For my reassurance Liza handed the cell phone to our *mamacita* and I spoke with her and reassured her she was going for a drive and I could almost imagine *mamacita* smiling. She expressed to me this very special smile when she was happy and I could almost see it and also heard her sweet voice. I have to confess, I must have called Liza at least 3–4 more times that night while she was on the road. Liza also told me they stopped several times for obvious reasons, hunger, bathroom, hunger and bathroom. Of course she verbalized to me the major problem, which was *¡EL CINTURON! (The SEAT BELT!) "The drive was a constant struggle, MOM DOES NOT LIKE BEING STRAPPED IN HER SEAT! Every time she would unbuckle her belt, I would manage to clip it back on right away and still stay focused on my driving, but with one eye on her. I had the radio on playing Spanish music, cantando como loca* (singing like crazy) but driving safely. I finally had enough of *peleando con el cinturon* (fighting with the seat belt) that when she unbuckled it for the umpteenth time, *me hize pendeja* . . . (I acted stupid) and I pretended I did not see her unbuckle it AGAIN. It was such an issue. I talked to God and asked him to help me out, and guide us home safely. I said, 'I put this in your hands.' That is something my mom would say; now I am saying it. We arrived home safely and quite late that night. What a full day!" It was a very long ride according to Liza, but she accomplished the mission and arrived in Houston, safely! *Gracias a Dios!* (Thanks be to God) Alleluia! Amen!

Upon their arrival Liza also told me *mamacita* was introduced to her grandchildren, who warmly welcomed her. I will now share *mamacita*'s life in Houston. This writing is with Liza's permission and in her own words:

"First time I cared for mom:" I had MOM under my care at my house and I thought it went well. She is my mother, and therefore part of my new *familia* (family), my own children and husband, and all the pets we have accumulated. It was no struggle to fit her into our lifestyle. I cared for mom at my house for what started to be two weeks, but stretched out into almost a month. I had a spare bedroom that we set up with familiar items of her house hoping that she would feel less scared in her new surroundings. On the wall, I hung family pictures. Of course, she brought her dog along. And of course, we had to bring the potty-chair. We traveled the four-hour drive from San Antonio to Houston without telling her where we were going. I would tell her that we were almost "there" when she would ask if we were going home. She finally figured out that we had been on the road for a long time; I could not fool her.

I stayed in her room most of the day and well into the night. I set up my laptop in her room so that I could work and still keep an eye on her. She liked to read. I remember once when she proudly announced to me that she was almost finished reading this one book, about Padre Pio. But

I realized that she would pick up the book and just start randomly reading from whatever page was open. I wonder how much of the book she did read, or if she remembers any of what she read. It was a good way to keep her occupied! Part of our daily routine was to walk the two long blocks to the elementary school at 3 P.M. in the afternoon to pick up my little daughter. We got our exercise that way. I would help her down a flight of stairs and then she would loop her arm around mine as we merrily walked to the school.

During the day, I would give her the broom to sweep, whether it be the kitchen or the driveway. She seemed to enjoy doing that and I did not mind the extra help in housekeeping. I remember an amusing situation. I am in the habit of leaving my bagged groceries on the floor, not immediately putting the dry goods away. I had bought a candy bar for my little daughter and it was in one of the bags. I was sure of it, but my daughter Sarah could not find it. Then it dawned on me to check in Grandma's pocket! There was the candy bar, and it was half-eaten too. I thought it was funny; my mom had sticky fingers. If she saw something, she would think that it belonged to her and that is how she explained it to me. From that day on, I looked in her drawers regularly to look for items that were missing from the house.

As far as taking care of her personal needs, I would stand in the shower with her and help her bathe. She did not like to bathe, so I often gave her sponge baths and got away with washing her hair in the kitchen sink. It seemed to help pass the day quicker by keeping the radio on in her room as I worked on my computer. I would often converse with her, commenting on some particular song, specially a love song. "Mom," I would say to her, "is there such a thing as true love?" Her answer was "bullshit, *caca de toro*"! Then we would both laugh hysterically. I would do this several times, as she could not remember what was said five minutes before. I loved repeating this funny scene. The Spanish radio station gave us a lot of entertainment. KA CU CA KA was the name, or something like that, I can't remember and she would make fun of how it sounded every time they made a station announcement. After all, our *mamacita*'s name was the nickname of CUCA. CACA CUCU, *que*? We broke out in more laughter together. My kids looked at us wondering what all the laughter was about. I managed to video tape her and my family interacting, laughing and singing. She explained to me how she got her nickname which I never knew. I never showed her the tape for fear that she would not remember and thus get angry because she could display anger like hell hath no fury. She showed her anger one day when a neighborhood boy bathed her dog, which just set her off in a flurry. We were all stunned! She calmed down after about an hour and eventually commented that she had bathed the dog herself outside with the water hose! We all went along with her version of the dog bath as she looked so proud of herself and we held back our giggles.

We shared some "memorable moments" that will stay with me and my daughters forever. I call one of these episodes the "WENDY'S trip." I dropped off my two girls and their grandma at Wendy's, and drove off across the parking lot to a nail salon, feeling like I needed some special attention all alone to myself, and to get some pampering, which is *"raro"* (rare). I felt so proud of my oldest *meja*, (daughter), as she walked away toward the entrance of the fast food place, everyone smiling, as she was holding her grandma's hand so confidently, but I think that grandma might have been holding onto her granddaughter's hand for dear life. I reassured them all that I would be close by, just a walking distance away. As I drove away from Wendy's, I glanced in my rear view mirror to see "the girls" walking, hand in hand, and smiling. They met up with me at the nail salon and had to sit and wait for me. Grandma would not sit still. She kept getting up off the couch in the waiting area. Every time the phone would ring, she would get up to try to answer it, but Valerie would stop her and distract her. "It's not our phone, grandma, you cannot answer it!" she would say. This went on several times; again, the same thing. Thank goodness that my daughters thought that it was funny; they had never experienced anything like this before. They thought that grandma was "silly" and funny. They were very good at distracting her with offerings from the candy dish, and getting her to sit down on that special massage chair. After my nails were done, we had grandma pick out a color for her nails. She picked out a gaudy pink, but we all admired her choice. She even bragged that she had nice hands and fingernails. *Muy orguyosa* (proud!) was my *madre*. We ventured next to the grocery store. It was the first time we used one of those whatchamacallit-go-carts. Grandma sat in it, while I walked alongside, controlling the levers on the handlebars. Ayyy, *Dios Mio* (Oh, dear Jesus!) It was a jerky ride for my mom. I got the giggles because my girls saw me struggling with the controls, and I wish someone had taken a video of us. Grandma did not complain much. No, wait, she always complains, but somehow we managed to black that part out of our memories of that grocery trip. My girls enjoyed the opportunity in getting to drive that cart into the grocery store from the parking lot. Only grandma could have provided them with that valid excuse to play with the "*carrito*" (car) and not get in trouble. About that Wendy's thing, my daughter said, "Oh mom, grandma was so paranoid of any men in the place! She kept saying that some man sitting near to us might attack her. But I would tell her, NO, grandma, it is okay. And then she kept wanting to go up to everyone as they walked by to ask them to take her home. NO, NO, grandma, we don't know those people, you can't ask them that! Oh gosh, MOM. I was getting embarrassed. But I did realize that a lot of people smiled at us. I think they could tell that we were taking care of grandma, cause she is old, they could tell, and we are kind of young and they offered to open the door for us when we left. That was cool."

Taking care of MOM was an adventure and an eye opener, it was. Not so much for me, but for my kids and husband. I found I needed to take "breaks" from my mom by asking whoever was available to watch her, so I could go to the bathroom or whatever I could think up as an excuse. This remark says it all, it is from my youngest daughter, Sarah: "MOM, how can you do it? I cannot stand being with her for five minutes, and you are with her all the time?" I just smiled, a different kind of smile, "Now you know why I asked for your help." I was starting to get used to having her in my home, when it came time for her to return to her house. I knew that she could not care for herself properly and it was difficult to reverse roles with my mother. I did not mind at all. My heart was sad for "*la cucaracita*" (the little roach which was her nickname). I could not keep her in my care for a longer period of time. We have fond memories of her visits, though. I am glad that I have some of it on tape.

Mamacita's Return to San Antonio, Texas:

After three weeks, it was time for my return to reality; to being a caregiver to *mamacita*. After speaking with my sister as to logistics, we concluded we both had conflicts. We concluded to coordinate *mamacita*'s drop-off and pick-up date and time and, to meet at the halfway point at a fast food restaurant. Well, here we go again, I thought! Another adventure of the lives of two crazy daughters *con nuestra mamacita* (with our mother). ¡Que tontereras! (What craziness), as *mamacita* would say. As we each started our drive, we called each other on the cell phone about every hour or so to learn of our location. To be quite honest, I felt really silly driving down the freeway to pick up *mi mamacita*. I wondered and assured myself this was not the first nor the last time any family would do such a silly thing. I also thought to myself, how lucky our *mamacita* was that we were doing something like this for her. For a quick moment, I even pretended that I was in a movie going down the freeway to pick up our *mamacita*. How silly of me! Yea! Two silly daughters driving down the freeway; me, from San Antonio and Liza, from Houston. Wow! What a coordinated job, what a BIG JOB! How silly of us. Oh well, my husband and I just laughed and smiled as we talked about our drive. How funny!

Two hours and 150 miles later, we all met at McDonald's in Columbus, Texas. When Liza stopped her Suburban, I rapidly walked over to see *mi mamacita*. When she saw me, she smiled and said, "*¿Tiengo hambre, me vas a llevar a mi casa?*" (I am hungry, are you going to take me home?) "*Por favor, llevarme a mi casa.*" ("Please, take me home.") I quickly thought, yep, this is the same *mamacita* I left a few weeks ago; she had not changed! Obviously, she has not missed me, oh well. She did not even say hello, how are you? How was your trip? No way, José. Well, *así es la vida* (that is life)! I grabbed her hand and we walked together to the restaurant. I bought *mamacita* some ice cream while Liza and my husband repacked from one car to the other.

Whew, finally, the packing was completed which included the potty-chair. To San Antonio we go! Here goes, I said to myself, gotta drive down the highway, just the three of us, *mamacita*, my husband and I. Great, this is going to be fun. *Me sentir contenta* (I felt happy) that my husband was a good person. He is the best, flexible, patient, honorable person to help me with my mother. Here we are on the road, with the Spanish CD, Vicente Fernández, on, and the three of us singing. How much happier can life be? Okay, are we one happy family or what? Within fifteen minutes of this beautiful drive down the freeway, I saw *mi mamacita* remove her seat belt. Can you believe it—and right in front of my eyes! I said to myself, hay ya, ya, here we go again; it is the seat belt problem AGAIN! I hurriedly asked *mi mamacita*, "Why did you remove your seat belt?" She said, "Estoy muy apretado, me siento como un marano." (It is too tight, I feel like a stuffed pig). I thought, oh dear Jesus, help me! *Mi mamacita* does not like the seat belt; she takes it off often and is removed many more times than it is on. Oh, mother, what am I going to do with you? I tried to distract her as I have always done but without success. Let me tell you, after the constant distractions, and reassurances of the safety factor, the drive back was very nervous for my husband and me.

After a half hour of this nerve-wracking scenario, my husband and I decided to stop for a break (another one of course). I looked into the back seat and was astonished and alarmed that *mi mamacita* was all tied up onto her own seat belt. She really did look like a "stuffed pig," to borrow her expression, but my husband and I could not believe what we saw. My husband and I concluded she had tried to remove her seat belt and somehow managed to get herself stuck between it. It was an unbelievable sight to see. My husband and I looked each other in amazement and tried not to laugh, but it really was funny. We quickly decided to find a solution to remove the seat belt because of the possible restriction of circulation to her extremities. My husband and I quickly and safely repositioned her down on her side and pulled her one leg out through the seatbelt and then the other. Finally, she was loose! Whew! What a relief! We three were so relieved! Alleluia! *Gracias a Dios*! (Thanks be to God!) One can only imagine trying to loosen up *mi mamacita* as she constantly said, "Get this XXXX seat belt off me, *me siento como un marano.*" (I feel like a stuffed pig.)

After this incident, we drove home without her seatbelts on, to say the least. I prayed to our *Dios* (our Lord) to help us have a safe drive. No more seat belt complaints, Amen. Finally, as the sun set, we arrived in San Antonio safe and sound! *Gracias a Dios* (Thanks be to God). My husband and I were both exhausted but ironically, *mi mamacita* was not. I could not believe I had difficulty convincing her of bedtime. Thanks to the nightfall, she convinced herself. She went to sleep without too much difficulty this time.

To this date, my husband still talks about that seat belt scenario. Of course, I spoke with my younger brother about this incident to see if he could come up with an extra seat belt or another solution and none was found. We continued to monitor and encourage *mi mamacita* not to take her seat belt off each trip we got in the car.

17

Adult Day Care
(*La Escuelita para Adultos*)

On one beautiful April spring day, after two long months of waiting, the phone finally rang! I felt this phone call was no ordinary call. This phone call came on a Thursday afternoon and what a wonderful day it was for me! On the other side of the phone I heard a female voice which identified herself from Grace Place Day Care. My heart stopped for a very brief moment, and speeded up with excitement. I thought, is this the call? The call for *mamacita* to go to Day Care? The soft-spoken woman on the other side of the phone told me that space was available for *mi mamacita* to attend Day Care starting the immediate next Monday. Hurrah! She also asked me if it would be possible for me to go the next day to sign the appropriate paperwork. Of course, I said YES! With excitement within me, I thanked her and literally and figuratively jumped for joy! Hurrah! Thanks be to God! (*Gracias a Dios!*) The Day Care acceptance for *mi mamacita* had finally arrived! Alleluia! Amen! *Mi mamacita* is going to Day Care, I said to myself! Thanks be to God! (*Gracias a Dios!*) I was so excited I immediately had to notify everyone! I was that excited! I told everyone, my husband, my younger brother, my younger sister, my sons and my friends. I also e-mailed the rest of the family about the happy news. This definitely was a very happy and joyous day in the life for *mi mamacita* and I. Sadly, I must say, I could not tell *mi mamacita* because she could not understand. Day Care is a new concept and I thought she might misunderstand the situation of sending her away; after all, she had seen only me, every day, for the past four months! In addition, she had never heard of Day Care, not even for children. I knew deep within my heart, there was no way possible for me to explain this to her NOW! No, I could not hurt her feelings. What for? Sometimes, one has to make the decision in protecting a loved one and not tell them everything. If you must tell them, tell them gently and in lesser amount of words; and of course, not that same day. Remember, they are very sensitive and can be hurt easily.

I am so excited to tell you about Adult Day Care! I can hardly wait to tell you! Interestingly, I too learned about this new concept and I learned fast. It is the same concept as a day care for children but quite different, because it is for adults, so their mission and programs are different. Adults like one's mother, father, aunt, uncle, and grandparent. WOW! I said! Adult Day Care, what a wonderful idea! This is fabulous! Having an Adult Day Care is a blessing whereby our beloved elderly family member can be dropped off at a safe and fun environment for a day or designated time period while the caregiver can go to work or do other responsibilities. Rest assured that it is a lifesaver! Let me tell you more about Adult Day Care. They have supervised programs that are fun and stimulating for them. At the same time, they serve good and nourishing food. Hmmm, good! This particular Day Care, Grace Place, is specialized with care of Alzheimer's clients. Double Hurrah! Their programs included activities that are changed every twenty minutes to continue to provide stimulation. Some of their activities/programs consist of:

- Bingo,
- Singing,
- Coloring,
- Exercising,
- Playing Ball,
- Playing Dominoes,
- Story telling/listening,
- Playing other types of games, for example: cutting coupons or drawing.[4]

Funny thing, though, I was told each client was a winner and the prize was a snack, how yummy! Wow! I like that kind of game! That is cute and smart of the staff! I am sure *mi mamacita* loved it and the other clients do too.
Other activities included:

- Beauty Shop day: Hairstyling and Mani-cures—(how beautiful-¡*hay, que bonitas*!)
- Watching TV,
- Field Trips to the mall and van rides.[4]

In regards to the food they eat, I had the opportunity to look at the menu selections, and noted the menu to be:

- Pork and Squash (*Calabasita*),
- Lasagna,
- Spaghetti,
- Arroz con Pollo, (Chicken with rice),
- Salisbury steak, Meatloaf, Seafood, and other yummy food,
- Of course, many more different kinds of good food (*papitas*, like my mother would say).

- Beverages, like milk, juices and ice tea; let me tell you, they did not go thirsty, but NO sodas! HURRAH! And they were very cautious with diabetic clients.[4] Hmm, it makes me hungry just writing about it! I can reassure everyone *mi mamacita* never complained about the food. After all, she loved to eat and most of the Alzheimer's clients loved to eat too.

Day Care Drop-off

I am so excited to tell you about *mi mamacita* and her first day at the Day Care. The first day I dropped her off, well, it was <u>most</u> invigorating for me! Yep, me, her daughter! First of all, I had to pre-plan her morning to a different schedule in order to drop her off at the opening time of 9 A.M. but unfortunately this time did not work. I guess I was just too slow and not organized enough to be there on time. I had to make many changes in my morning schedule in order to adjust to *mi mamacita* and rightly so. I have to admit, I did not accomplish dropping her off on time because I miscalculated the time it would take me to get my eighty-two-year-old *mamacita* who happens to have arthritis. Oh, dear Jesus (*hay Jesusito*). Within two days though, I learned to accomplish the routine and dropped her off by 11:30 A.M. Hurrah! Now, that is an accomplishment, if you ask me. I do know that I had to learn to get myself and her on a faster routine, I am sure I would learn. Oh, well, here goes Day Care. Timidly, I must admit, I felt like a mother of a young child. Everything about getting her ready for Day Care made me reminisce of my sons (*de mis hijos*). It was like "déjà vu"; quite a flashback. From getting *mamacita* dressed in a pretty dress, shoes and socks to match, to ensuring that she had her teeth brushed. It is amazing how the world turns. I was a mother again, but differently! WOW! But yes, I was excited for her. I made it a practice not to tell her in advance, because she would not understand and I just told her each time we were going "bye-bye." I honestly believe she must have known something was going on because she readily got dressed without difficulty. Whew! Okay, we are dressed now, finally. While holding hands, we walk together to the car. We get into the car, I turn on the Vicente Fernandez CD, and away I drove to the day care as we both sing, La, La, La, La. After a fifteen minute drive, *mamacita* and I arrived at the Day Care parking lot. I got off and told her, "Come on, *mamacita*, we are going to visit some friends." I put my hand out and she grabs it. We walk together to the building door and the staff sees me and *mi mamacita* and they open the door and grabbed *mi mamacita* from me while saying, "Good Morning, Mary, how are you?" *Mi mamacita* dramatically grabs my hand and said, "You are not leaving me here!" ("¡*Tu no me vas a dejar aqui!*") Firmly but gently, I said, "Yes, *mamacita*, I need to go to work, I will be back to pick you up." I turned around, go out the door and they gently guide her in. I did not look back. I did not see *mi mamacita* that day until 4:30 P.M. when I picked her up and I did not call the Day Care, I was at peace; *mi mamacita* was in good hands.

That afternoon, upon my arrival, I saw my *mamacita*'s smile and her lips moving as she walked to the glass door. As the Day Care door opened, *mi mamacita*'s smile got bigger and she said, "I am so happy that you are picking me up, I was waiting for you." I too smiled and told her that I too was happy to see her! I grabbed her hand and we walked together to the car and asked her how her day was. She replied, "It was nice." I also asked her, "What did you do today?" She responded, "We colored," or another day she said, "Today we played some games," or "They painted my nails, look, aren't they pretty?" She said these proudly while smiling continuously as she told me about her day. I am proud to say that it was beautiful to see her being happy as well as a welcome relief that she likes Day Care. It took *mi mamacita* about four LONG months to finally settle into the new routine of going to Day Care. Of course, I cannot fully understand what she really thinks but I do know she is happy because she answers YES and with a smile on her pretty face. Oh yes, *mi mamacita* and I have a very interesting kind of relationship. I am most happy to have been given the opportunity to provide Day Care for her. In the past, one could never imagine *mi mamacita* would have gone to Day Care. NEVER! (*NUNCA!*) It was not around, not even in anybody's mind. Today, we live very different lives. Wow! Our parents in Day Care? Wow! Anyway, I had no problems with the idea. In fact, I strongly recommend it, for their sake, as well as the caregiver. Yea!

It was now time for "Show and Tell." Story time: Yes, *mi mamacita* came home with "Goodies" too. She was so cute! SMILE! These stories will bring back memories to those of you who are parents of young children. Remember, those days when your children (*cuando tu niños*) went to Day Care? Nice memories, right? (For example, a coloring book page, a gift box or a note as a reminder of pick-up time. Interestingly, I too have found some of these notes in some unbelievable places on *mi mamacita* (in her bra, socks and even in her underwear). Oh, mother! (*Hay, mamacita!*) I chuckle with the excitement that I really have to check her clothes thoroughly upon her return each day. Also, for those special occasions, she came home with a picture, for example, Birthday, Christmas, Fiesta or Mother's Day. The Day Care really tried to keep the clients orientated as to time, and also to keep them happy and occupied. Go for it, Day Care. Hurrah!

Here are some samples of the Day Care activities:[4]

Sample of Letter to Pick Her Up:

Mother,
Iwill pick
you up today at
4:00 pm
be good and
have fun.

love you,
Mary Teresa

Sample of Activity

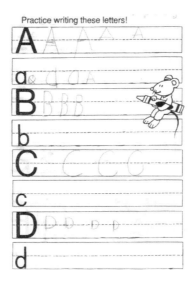

Practice writing these letters!

A A A A A A

a a a a A

B B B B

b

C C C C C

c

D D D D D

d

18

Special Occasions
(*Ocasiónes Especiales*)

Happy Birthday (*Feliz Cumpleaños*):

In this chapter for fun, I am sharing some family occasions to tell everyone, **yes**, one can still have family times; just individualize them. Here are some listed specifically: *mamacita's* birthday; Valentine's Day, Fiesta, Easter, Mother's Day, family contributions, Thanksgiving Day and Christmas.

In January 2000, I started a celebration custom for my mother's eightieth Birthday. It was so much fun that I have continued this for *mi familia* (our family) to celebrate and thank my dear God for *mi mamacita*! For me, part of the fun was the preparation; just like Christmas and Thanksgiving. I am sure that some of you are saying, fun? I know, for some, it is fun, while for others, it is work. I have learned that one must enjoy our parents and families because one does not know what our future holds in store for us. So enjoy!

My party plans included advance planning and notifying *mi familia* including date and time as well as the menu: (see next pages 176–177)

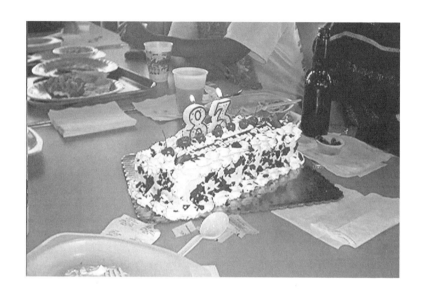

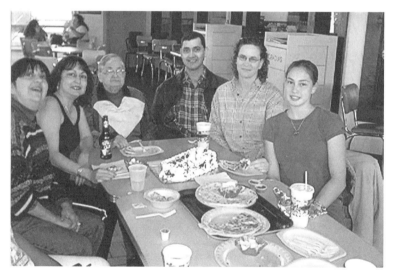

Our Party Menu:

- Tamales
- Frijoles—la charra (whole, in liquid)
- Potato Salad
- Arroz (rice)
- Chips (several kinds)
- Guacamole & cheese dip
- Sodas (various kinds)
- Cerveza (beer)

I asked *mi familia* for their suggestions, contributions and for their confirmation of attendance. I also called my younger brother who lived in San Antonio for his assistance in ordering the *Mariachis.*

The Party Day Arrived (*Llego el día*):

Let's go shopping for the party everybody! I know, you are probably wondering, why shopping? What are they going to buy? Now, don't tell me they are buying store-bought food? Did I say store-bought food? Good question! One might probably ask, why don't they just cook it like it used to be in my *costumbre* (custom)? Well let me tell you, home-cooked food is much better but, I must explain. Please, oh please, let me explain. No, I am not making excuses for myself, but I did have to fly across the country for this party and its preparations, what can I say? Also, most of us lived out of town, on time crunches, and running around like "chickens without heads." I have concluded, we just had to satisfy ourselves with store-bought food and fix it up a little bit. I learned how to spice up the *frijoles* (pinto beans) or any other food by adding my own personal touches! (Smells good to me!) Come on now, can you smell the fresh *frijoles*, arroz (rice), and the *tamales* as they are cooking on the stove? Hmm . . . just don't tell our *mamacita* it is store-bought food, I won't! Yea, store-bought food is better than NO food. Sorry about that! *Así es la vida! (That is life!)*

I sure miss *mi mamacita*'s home cooking as she does not cook anymore. I feel sad when I think how Alzheimer's has robbed *mi mamacita* and my family of the treasures of cooking. Wow! She used to cook the most delicious *frijoles,* and *arroz* and potato salad. I am sorry that she did not develop the talent to cook *tamales,* but she was very, very busy with nine children and I cannot blame *mi mamacita* for this, anyway. *Hay caramba!* (Oh, my goodness!) I am sure that at least one of you knows someone who cooks *tamales* as a tradition every year. Not us, though, we satisfied ourselves with the factory *tamales.* We were blessed to have plenty around in San Antonio. Hurrah! Hmmm, they were good. Whatever works for each family is all that matters!

Llego el Party (Party Time has Arrived):

It is six in the evening and the *Mariachis* have arrived at the front gate. Hurrah! Party time! We could hear them singing and playing the song, *Las Mananitas,* (the birthday song) as they strolled up the sidewalk. Oh, how beautiful, I thought. I wish everyone could have seen *mi mamacita*'s eyes sparkle and the gleam in her beautiful big smile! This definitely was a very special moment. There were no words to explain, just smiles to try to explain. We all knew these moments as "Kodak moments."

178

(I give credit for this.) Thanks for letting me borrow these words.

Oh, how beautiful. . . .

Please sit down on a chair, close your eyes and take a deep breath and try to imagine the *Mariachis* playing for you for one whole hour of your favorite Mexican songs. Now, that is a winner! Enjoy them! After all, that is exactly what I did. I do have to brag, these Mexican songs along with the family sing-alongs were "LIVE" in *mi mamacita*'s living room as my family enjoyed these happy moments. To my great surprise, my mother was singing these songs in Spanish. Did I say, *mi mamacita* was singing? Yes, *mi mamacita* was singing! *Hay caramba!* (Oh my goodness!) I have witnessed a beautiful thing and so my friends, I am a lucky girl! *¡Gracias a Dios!* (Thanks to God!)

For your enjoyment, here are the names of some of our favorite Mexican songs which were played at that beautiful birthday party. Maybe you too, can enjoy them in your mind. I am sure there are many more songs out there. Maybe, you can take a few minutes and try to remember your favorite songs. Please don't stress yourself thinking though. Remember, you are suppose to relax and enjoy. So enjoy!

Mexican Songs (*Canciónes Mexicanas*):

- Volvér, Volvér (Return, Return)
- Creé (I believed)
- Un Rincón en una Cantina (A corner in a bar)
- Gabino Barrera (A name of a Mexican drunk man)
- Un Caballo Blanco (A white horse)
- Un Caballo Negro (A black horse)

- Mejico (Mexico)
- Margarita, Margarita (Margaret, Margaret)
- El Rey (The king)
- Las Mananitas (The birthday song)
- Jalisco (Name of a city in Mexico)
- La Cucaracha (The cockroach)
- Un Reloj (The watch)
- La Bamba (The band)
- El Rancho Grandé (The large ranch)
- El Caballo Prieto (The dark horse)
- Sin Teé (Without you)

Here is a picture of the Mariachis playing:

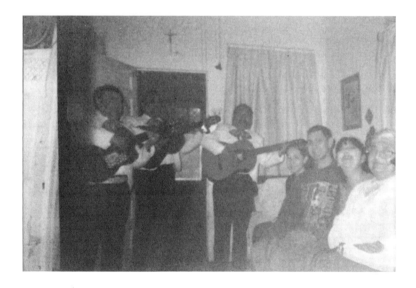

Personal Suggestions

If you decide to order *Mariachis* for your loved one's *cumpleaños* (birthday), make sure and shop around because they play and charge by the hour. (Some groups have a large number of singers in the group so the price goes up). Also, for your convenience, make sure that a written list of the songs is made because an hour is a long time. I chuckle today, for us, we ran out of songs and had a heck of a time trying to recall other songs. I guess we had a lapse of memory but we still had a lot of fun anyway!

Valentine's Day (*Día de Valentinos*)

Another happy occasion for us was Valentines Day. Happy Valentine's Day to everyone, especially those of you who take care of your loved ones. In 2002, I am happy to report *mi mamacita* received phone calls, greeting cards and flowers by a couple of family members. I, on behalf of our *madrecita,* would like to thank them and may God bless them. **Happy Valentine's Day!**

I will end this tribute with one of my mother's *dichos*:
While young, it's all dreams; when old, all memories. [2]
(*Cuando joven, de ilusiones; cuando vieja, de recuerdos, de recuerdos.*)

Fiesta Is Alive (¡*Viva Fiesta!*)

Let me first try to explain what **FIESTA** is all about in San Antonio, Texas. It is an annual event which celebrates Texas' independence from Mexico, because at that time, Texas was part of Mexico. This battle occurred in the city of San Jacinto, Texas on April 21, 1836. Personally, I think that is why we Texans continue to celebrate this anniversary for the past 100 years and continue to do so to this day every year. In other words, another reason to party! Fiesta is ten days of fun, fun, fun! It is like a Mardi Gras which occurs in New Orleans, Louisiana. It occurs on the third week of April, every year, and the whole city celebrates. It is a holiday for the school children and the businesses close at twelve noon on Fiesta Friday for families to enjoy the parade and have fun too.

The Fiesta celebrations are kicked off with a river parade on the first Monday. The parade consists of beautiful, colorful barges and filled with music caroling in the air from around the world. Other fun activities include: a carnival, a band festival, a Queen coronation and two kings, King Antonio and *Rey Feo* (the ugly king). These two kings visit the local elementary schools and the hospitals and bring the children warm cheer and joy. They also raise money for children's scholarships. Included in these festivities are the local and out of town schools, universities and civic organizations who join in the celebration by providing entertainment, food and arts/crafts throughout the whole week. Hurrah! Party time!

The Fiesta celebrations are climaxed with a Battle of Flowers Parade on Friday afternoon and with the Fiesta Flambeau on Saturday night. These parades are absolutely spectacular with the flowers, lights, dignitaries, clowns, local city government, balloons and much, much more. The parade consists of national school bands, universities, the military and civic organizations and the opportunity to show off their colors and their pride. It is a wonderful city-wide celebration! These celebrations give hundreds of tourists the opportunity to have some fun and wonderful memories. If you ever get the opportunity, come on down to San Antonio, Texas on the third week of April. Be prepared to have some great South Texas fun! You all come now, you hear!

My story will now focus on the Fiesta Day Care Party because everyone in San Antonio has a Fiesta Party which include Day Care too! Yes they do! One day, I was so surprised when *mi mamacita* came home with a Fiesta party invitation for clients and families. Hurrah! Fiesta party! We both smiled as I read it out loud. Of course, my first thought was, a dress. Hmm, you probably are saying, just like girls, they need a dress. Yep, you are correct, because this is the only time whereby it is OK to dress up in Fiesta apparel which have ruffles, ribbons, bows and flowers. The men wear a *Guayabera* (a Mexican style shirt) with comfortable slacks.

Well, I thought, before we go shopping we have to look in the closet; I was sure that a festive dress was around somewhere. After all, we attend fiesta celebrations every year. I decided to look in the closet by playing games, after all, *mi mamacita* loves to play games. We played peek-a-boo and hide and seek. She laughed and smiled as we both had a lot of fun looking for a dress. We looked and looked and finally found some clothes for both of us little party girls. Hurrah!

Day Care Fiesta Has Arrived (*Lelego el día de el Fiesta Party del Day Care*)

Let me tell you, *mi mamacita* and I were very excited about this party. This day, she did not mind taking a bath; she must have sensed the excitement in my voice. I bathed and dressed her first. (I remembered when my sons were young and I dressed them last, I was always dirty or wet before them). (Chuckle.) So now, I dress *mamacita* first! I dressed her in a bright pink Mexican dress which had ruffles and beautiful, large multi-colored flowers and I put a ribbon in her hair, a beaded necklace and some matching earrings. We were both excited as was confirmed in the mirror. To top the beauty of it all, she even asked for lipstick which I applied excitedly. I sat her down on a chair and told *mi mamacita* it was my turn to get dressed and told her to watch television and wait for me. I cannot believe I said that because I must have had a senior moment or something, for *mi mamacita* to wait, no way, José! Because I just heard her saying, "Terry, I am dressed, are we going to the party?" I guess I too have a short memory to forget that *mi mamacita* had no patience. I dressed in a hurry, of course. Ironically, she kept saying, "*Que pokey*" (How slow you are). I just smiled.

Finally I was dressed! I would hardly believe my ears if *mi mamacita* would have said, "About time!" Of course, *mi mamacita* looked prettier than me, but I too looked pretty, I might add. I am sure *mi mamacita* and I were a walking advertisement for Fiesta. Chuckle. . . . Go Fiesta! For a quick moment, I thought about the storybook tale that goes something like this: "Mirror, mirror on the wall, who is the prettiest of them all?" (I give credit due.) *Mi mamacita,* of course, is the prettiest of them all! Oh, well, I am proud of *mi mamacita.* Finally, we were dressed and we walked to the car, smiling, and I drove to the Day Care which was about fifteen minutes away. All along the drive *mi mamacita* asked, when are we getting to the party? No matter how many times I answered her, she repeated these same words. I told *mi mamacita* we were almost there but she smiled and repeated these same words. Oh dear Lord, please give me patience, I thought.

Upon our arrival to the Day Care, we were greeted by the staff who also were dressed up. The Day Care was festively decorated with a large-starred piñata, Fiesta posters and brightly colored paper-maché flags. WOW! How festive! We both smiled! We were told to wait and play games while the piñata was filled with candy as is my custom. Afterwards, we were guided to the main dining room to join the rest of the clients with their families to play games. *Hay, que cute* (Oh, how cute).

One of the games the clients played was an exercise game. A musical tape cassette was started and described how to play. It was real cute, it went like this: take your right hand out, bring it up into the sky and shake it all about, now put it down. Take your left hand out . . . and so forth and so on. I too joined in the exercise game just for the fun of it. One time, I even looked around at the other clients to see if they were following directions and to my amazement, they were. I was so impressed and almost shocked they were all coordinated. Wow! Of course, I was stunned and pleased to see my *mamacita* following directions too. I thought, wow, *mi mamacita* following directions, wow! I can't believe my eyes, I guess seeing is believing! She even caught me seeing her and I smiled. We also played ball together. There was a large beach ball which was thrown to each other and in return to another person. This game was kind of fun too.

I tried to leave my *mamacita* alone so I could see her interaction with the other clients but she would not let me out of her sight. At one time, I got out of my chair and she said, *"No te vayas"* (do not leave). I was stunned in my shoes. After awhile, it got amusing because, I moved away from her onto another chair and she followed me.

Interestingly, I thought she felt secure with me and did not want me to leave; basically she was glued to me. I also tried to encourage her to participate in the group activities and she would not. This reminded me of her being "*chiflada*" ("spoiled"). Well, of course as a stubborn daughter, I was determined to accomplish my mission, that of watching her interaction with others. I thought, Hmm, I have to come up with a plan. Light bulb turned on, I decided to go to the bathroom. I got up from my chair and said, "*Voy al baño, horita vengo para atras.*" (I am going to the bathroom, I will return.) She looked at me and said, "Okay." I quickly walked away toward the bathroom and then stopped around the corner and I continued to see her. I then saw her coloring, singing and eating a snack. I was pleased with what I saw. This proved to me that she was adjusting to her new environment, the Day Care. Hurrah! Thank you, Jesus! (*¡Gracias!*)

Piñata time (*Llego tiempo para la piñata*):

Suddenly a loud bell rang along with a verbal announcement that it was party time and it was time to break the piñata. We were instructed to form a single line, which we all did excitedly (just like in school, how cute we looked)! We walked outside together, *mi mamacita* and I, as we smiled and obeyed orders. As soon as we arrived into the outside patio, we all saw a giant brightly colored Star Piñata which was hanging on a rope. I observed two staff members holding it and also smiling. Several clients eyes gleamed and exclaimed, "*Que bonita la piñata*" (what a beautiful piñata). The staff then asked each client, including *mi mamacita*, to get into a line to hit the piñata. As each client hit the piñata, the crowd roared

186

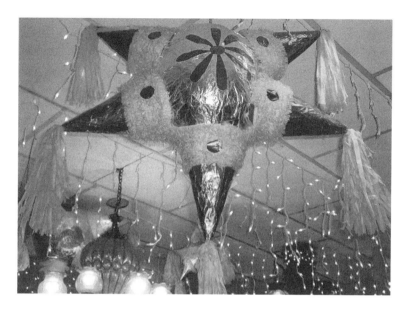

La Piñata

and none broke it this particular time. It was *mi mamacita*'s turn. She turned her face and looked at me for approval and I said, "Go, *mamacita*, go hit the piñata." Like a child, she did not hesitate. With all her energy, she hit the piñata three times as was the limit for each client and she too could not break it. A staff member finally broke the piñata and divided the candy among all of the clients. It was cute to see all the clients get out of their chair and run with excitement to get candy. I thought, wow, they really are having fun, just like children. Amazing!

It was so much fun to see them have a good time at the piñata game. What can I say, they deserve to have fun too. After the piñata game, we all marched back into the dining room for cake and punch. Hmm, that was delicious. After the cake, the party was over and we all went home. I talked about this party to *mi mamacita* for the rest of the afternoon, but of course, I had to remind her that we actually went to a Fiesta Party because she could not believe me. Oh, well, I was happy we both had a good time but at the same time, sorry that she could not remember five minutes after we left the party. *Hay, que vida!* (That is life!)

Easter (*Día de Pascua*):

My memories of Easter have to date before my mother had Alzheimer's because currently, we do not celebrate Easter with her. I have concluded there are too many problems in trying to organize my family members and for many other reasons beyond my control. I did decorate my condominium with Easter bunnies but *mamacita* did not understand this special date. She continued to receive flowers and greeting cards from some *familia* (family).

As a child, let me assure you, Easter at my parents' home was a very happy and blessed occasion. Okay, here comes memory lane, please bear with me. I remember *mamacita* ensuring that we were well-dressed. It was like she took it upon herself to show us off and all of us children had nice, new clothes to go to church. The girls wore frilly dresses with matching shoes, purse and hat. The boys wore a suit. I still remember that beautiful red chiffon dress with a white bib on it. I looked so cute. I honestly believe special occasions were the only times we had new clothes. We were blessed!

On the next page is one of her fond memories of Easters when she was a child:

Pink is my
favorite color.
I like to wear
1 or 2 pink
dresses. I
had a light
green dress
for easter when
I was a little girl!

I would take
my Easter
basket to church
waiting for the
mass to finish
then we would
have the easter
egg hunt. It was
very exceiting. I
liked the candy.

I do not like
Cascarones eggs.
However, I did
like the chocolate
Bunnies that my
mother gave to
me for easter.
When we were
small we would

go to church.
There were
beautiful pink
easter flowers
in church. They
took them outside.
The church had
easter egg hunts
when I was a
little girl. I had
a big family.

Oh, well, enough dreaming for me, I have to go back to work. Hmm. It was very traditional to go to church as a family, including my dad. After church, we went on a picnic and had an Easter egg hunt. Oh yea, that was real fun too, running around like a treasure hunt and trying to get the most eggs. I remember breaking these *cascarones* (eggs filled with confetti) on my brother's heads because we loved doing that and we just laughed. I do have to admit, the preparation for the egg hunt was the best part of this fun activity. I remember *mi mamacita* saved egg shells and egg whites for at least two-three months for the Easter egg hunts. The day before Easter, *mi mamacita* taught us how to dye these shells with different color dyes, like, yellow, purple, green, red . . . oh, how pretty they all looked. We were so thrilled and excited we could not wait for the Easter Sunday egg hunt.

Mother's Day (*El Día de Las Madres*):

Feliz Día de Madres (Happy Mother's Day) to all mothers and caregivers in our world. May God or whomever they worship bless them!

On this very beautiful day it always gives me the opportunity to think of the memories of *mi mamacita* and what she means to me. There are tributes everywhere, on television, in newspapers, schools, etc. I would like to share a tribute to all the mothers in the whole world! I would also like to thank all of *mi mamacita*'s children and grandchildren who have remembered her throughout her life. Most especially these past few years when *mamacita* has needed it the most. Thank you and may God bless you!

Okay, everybody, sit down, take a deep breath and enjoy this tribute to all the *mamacitas*. This special day started with a Mass at the local church with *Mariachis,* of course. Please imagine hearing *Mariachis* playing a beautiful song called, *Las Mañanitas* (The morning). After church, we went to eat at a restaurant and guess what we saw? More *Mariachias!* Now, try to listen to another Mexican song. We went to the cemetery, guess again, more *Mariachis.* The cemetery looked beautiful with flowers everywhere. The cemetery, one might wonder? I need to explain about going to the cemetery on this special day in my Hispanic(Latin) custom. Well, it is a custom showing respect to our deceased mothers, grandmothers and all the female relatives. *Mariachis* is a custom also. How beautiful! This day in my culture is a VERY IMPORTANT day! It is so important because mothers are a "gift" from God. In other words, in my religion, Jesus too had a mother and he loved her very much.

To conclude this tribute, I decided to ask my family for their personal experiences or thoughts about *mamacita* and what she means to them. Here are a few that I received. I dedicate all of them to our *mamacita.* Please remember, these are for your reading pleasure, so smile if you like. Hello there, maybe these too will refresh some good memories *de tu mamacita* (of your mother), so smile and enjoy!

- My mother is beautiful,
- Her laughter is stupendous; it shines like the sky,
- My mother helped me grow up,
- My mother was there when I needed her,
- When I was small, my mother bought me a dress, shoes, purse, and hat every Easter,
- My mother loved all of her children even though she sometimes did not show it,
- My mother breast fed me when I was a baby,
- My mother showed me how to pray,

- My mother gave me a lot of presents,
- My mother gave me candies,
- My mother gave me kisses,

Other Family Contributions (from Her Daughter, Sylvia)

"I remember most of *mi mamacita* were her funny faces. She always tried to make us kids laugh. I remember one specifically, when she would loosen her dentures and tried to scare us. She would walk around the room and go like a monster and we would all laugh. When she opened her mouth, the dentures would fall out. We all just laughed. My mother would always try to entertain us kids with her funny faces. She had that special motherly trait of making 'funny faces.' To this date I amusingly add, our *mamacita* continues to show us funny faces."

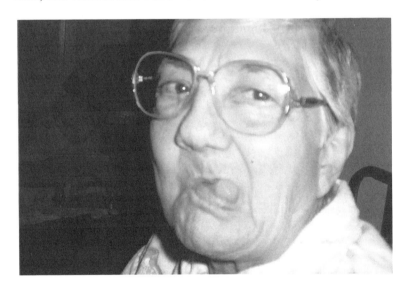

Mi mamacita's funny face

From Her Son, Tony

"I remember when my mother would chase me around the house and tried to say that she was going to cure me with an enema because I was always complaining of a stomach ache. You see, I would love to eat. She would approach me and say, 'Are you sick, my son, let me give you an enema.' I would run and run. No way was I going to get an enema. My mother was always giving me that Baby Percy and Castor Oil stuff. Ugh! I knew my mother too well! These memories of my mother while I was growing up have refreshed my relationship with her presently."

From Her Daughter, Liza

"I do not remember how old I was, but I must have been young since I do not remember any siblings being around to watch over me. My mom used to like to take a nap during the day and she had a special trick that she used on me so that she could sleep without worrying about me getting into any trouble. She would hand me a hairbrush and let me DO her hair. So, I would play with her hair, creating all kinds of different hair styles. Sometimes, she would wake up with braids, pony tails, and bobby pins carefully placed in strategic places all over her head but only on one side as she lay there peacefully sleeping. I bet she was surprised at what a good job I did and playing beauty shop on her! I never left her side as she slept because I was anxious to get praised for my newest hairstyle that I had given her. She sure kept me from getting into trouble. I stayed focused on her hair and had no desire to wander the house. Also, I credit my mother for nurturing my creativity. When I showed an interest in sewing, she always made sure that a sewing machine was available. For me, I started out sewing with a needle then of course a toy one and progressed to a real Singer sewing machine. She helped guide me with my natural talent. I appreciate how she helped me and I learned from her example. I also have paid attention to any special talents that my children possess and have tried to guide them to fully express that ability. I guide them and let them make their own decisions as my mother did with me. Thank God for a mother like her. I remember the time that my mother said, your hair looks like *te lambio una vaca* (a cow licked your hair), when my hair was not quite right. I still remember that no cows will ever lick my hair because I always check it before I leave the house. Thanks MOM, no cow will ever lick my head!"

From Her Granddaughter, Debbie

"When I was living with her and going to school half days, she would always have a can of spinach waiting for me so I could eat it while watching *Popeye*. This was very important to me then and she never forgot! She always let me hang around her at the house and let me help make dinner. She never got tired of me around her and never chased me off. We used to take bus rides downtown together to go shopping for nothing, just to be together. We laughed a lot too, she is my MOM. . . . All my good growing up memories as a kid are with Mom and Dad. Not that every day with Dad and Mom was perfect either, it wasn't sometimes, but you knew you were loved. I missed that the most growing up. Still do. Deb."

From Her Granddaughter, Karen

"My name is Karen and I grew up in San Antonio, Texas. I was one of many grandchildren of Mary and Reyes Schultz. I have fond memories of our large family coming together every Sunday afternoon after church. We always had a Bar-B-Q and I could count on Grandma to have a kitchen smelling of fresh cooked *arroz*, ranchero beans and homemade *tortillas de Harina*. I looked forward to skating in the backyard that grandpa had paved with concrete—a place grass couldn't grow because of all the kids. The men would gather together and have a couple of beers while the *fajitas* were cooking and the women would be cackling like hens around the small kitchen table in the house.

"I remember my grandmother recounting the week's events and telling of the new family gossip. She spoke in a Tex-mex style—a few words in Spanish, then a few in English—then in Spanish again. I always bugged my mom to translate for me because I couldn't ever get the whole story. I also remember Grandma's faithfulness to the local Catholic church, her many visits to help people in need whether they were family or not. She was always talking about Jesus—in fact, I am a Christian believer now and I know that it was through my Grandmother's devotion to her faith that the very first seeds of knowing about Christ's love was planted.

"There are a number of reasons why I believe we as a family need to help care and provide for our aging parents and grandparents. First and foremost, we should do it out of love, respect and reciprocity. We're all very busy and have our own families to care for. We no longer geographically live 'just down the street.' Despite these facts, we as a family and society have a moral obligation to provide for family members in need."

I conclude this beautiful chapter on our *mamacita* by sharing one more memory by child #8 as follows:

Memorias de Mi Madre—Memories of My Mother

"I was asked to write down some memories of our mom and I quickly said—Sure! But I struggle to try to condense a lifetime of my mom and me into a few short paragraphs or even a few pages. She is worth a book full of memories. She raised nine children, I raised six. I find my life is similar to hers. While growing up, a girl's worst nightmare was to be like YOUR MOM! I now see the legacy continues with my own daughters.

"Things my mom did: When I wanted to date a boy, she is the one who covered for me because my dad was a bit strict about it. She is a mother all through my adult life is what I remember. I cannot remember when I was little but seeds must have been planted already. When I had a problem, I would call MOM. She would console me. Never said anything negative. *Diocito sabe todo* (God knows everything), believe in God *'El' te ayuda* (HE will help you), she would say to me. Mom had special powers. I could call her or phone her when one of my kids was ill and I didn't know what to do. I unloaded on her, cried on her shoulder, complained to her and amazingly right after that, things got better. I always credited her with some special powers. She had a connection to a higher being! That is my mother!"

One more special memory, I just have to share these special words from *mi hermanita*, Liza. One day, because

I forgot what day it was, she told me, Happy Mother's Day. Now, that is something to smile about, to have Mothers Day *every day*! Hurrah! Smile!

If each one of you readers would like, you can write down or think of memories of your mother. Please do! I can almost bet a million dollars (if I had them) that a lot of people have a special memory of their mother as one was growing up. Happy Mother's Day to everyone!

Thanksgiving Day (*Día de Dar Gracias*)

Traditionally, this day is the day to give thanks for our material or spiritual goods. I thank God for *mi mamacita*, my husband and my sons, all of *mi familia* and my life. Throughout my life and before my mother acquired Alzheimer's, *mi familia* enjoyed beautiful family holidays. We also have been blessed to spend time together in my parents' home for Thanksgiving Day. In those days, *mi mamacita* cooked a grand dinner. Hmmm . . . it sure was delicious! I hope that you too have fond memories of Thanksgiving holidays.

Thanksgiving Day for *mi familia* has changed drastically as one can imagine. For about the past twenty years, *mi mamacita* has not cooked, and we managed to go to my parents' home before my father died and still have a family dinner. Some of her daughters took turns to cook the turkey while the rest of the family brought the other trimmings. As I mentioned earlier, we had wonderful family gatherings.

It is presently extremely difficult for my *familia* to truly enjoy any of the holidays. Alzheimer's has robbed *mi mamacita* and her family of the ability to enjoy life. I remember very well how our *mamacita* was the center of attention like a lot of mothers are and rightfully so. She was multi-talented like most *mamacitas* are. She was the chef, caregiver, maid, consoler, cook and bottle washer among many other job descriptions one can think of. That is life! As in my Hispanic/Latino culture, we all gathered in my parents' home for all the holidays. Those were the happy days.

As part of preparation for this beautiful day, I informed *mi familia* (per e-mail and phone calls) of the plans and asked them for their suggestions. Some of the family responded and some didn't. We had the party anyway because I wanted to make Thanksgiving Day special for *mi mamacita*. On the day before Thanksgiving, my husband, son and I flew to Texas for the Thanksgiving festivities.

Here are some stories of how we spend Thanksgiving Days before and after I moved to Texas. These are three very different stories as we tried to adjust to the circumstances of *mi mamacita*'s Alzheimer's. I must err on caution because only I and a few of *mi familia* were able to enjoy these holidays and accept *mamacita*'s Alzheimer's. It is extremely difficult for *mi familia* to truly enjoy any of these holidays but please try to remember she is still my *mamacita* and it is still Thanksgiving, sadly, though, quite different!

Thanksgiving Day (*Día de Dar Gracias*) (Before 24/7 Care)

Finally, Thanksgiving Day 2002 arrived and all of the family present were in a festive mood. My husband, sons and I spend the night at my brother's house so I could wake up early to cook the turkey. Several hours later, hmm . . . I smelled the turkey. Boy did it smell delicious. I could smell the aroma and could almost taste it! WOW! I announced with a excitement, the turkey is ready! I called *mi mamacita* on the telephone and told her that I was on the way to pick her up for dinner. I thought it might be easier to take *mi mamacita* over to his house instead of having all of the family go to her small house. I was definitely aware that *mi mamacita* did not like strange crowds. Upon my arrival to her house, I noted *mi mamacita* was not properly dressed. She was still wearing her pajamas at 2 P.M. in the afternoon. I bathed her and helped her into some appropriate clothes. Then my husband drove us to my brother's house. As I was dressing her, she kept asking, "*A donde vamos?*" (Where are we going?) I told her we were going to eat turkey at her son's house. She excitedly said, "*Pues muy bien, yo tiengo mucho hambre*" (well, that is good because I am real hungry).

During the thirty minute drive to Tony's house, *mamacita* smiled and repeated the same question at least ten times: "*¿A donde vamos?*" (Where are we going?) Each time, I answered her, "We are going to your son's house to eat turkey." Upon arrival to my brother's house, we all walked in together. Suddenly, after barely walking into the door and without notice, *mi mamacita* asked, "*¿A donde vamos?*" (Where are we going?) I told her again that we were at her son's house and she just smiled. I walked her to my brother, wife and nieces who greeted her warmly and they walked her to the living room to visit with the children. The other adults went to the kitchen to complete the dinner arrangements. I proceeded to set the table and through the corner of my eye, I saw the children fussing trying to entertain *mi mamacita*. My nieces were talking in a loud tone of voice and unsuccessfully trying to

199

distract *mi mamacita*. Upon seeing this, I called out, *"Mamacita, venga para la cocina, me puede ayudar aqui por favor?"* (Mother, please come to the kitchen, would you like to help me please?) Like a beautiful obedient child, *mi mamacita* immediately stood up and showed a big smile on her face and marched herself to the kitchen. I asked her to help me set the table which she gladly obliged. I felt that this was a simple task to ask of her that she could do successfully. The rest of the family were relieved that she helped readily. After all of the food was completed, I announced, "Dinner is ready, let's sit down!"

We all stood around the table and said prayers. We got into a line to serve ourselves our food, buffet style. I am proud to say, *mi mamacita* looked like an angel. She was smiling and appeared happy to be among her *familia* (family). It was a nice, happy and festive family gathering this Thanksgiving Day. Please note, I served her first to ensure she was kept busy. Suddenly, I saw a family member serving himself turkey and its trimmings and *mi mamacita* instantly rose from her chair and cut into the line. In a loud tone of voice, she said, *"¿Que estas haciendo con mi comida"* (What are you doing with my food?) along with a few cuss words, XXX. I quickly rose from my chair and in a soft-toned voice, gently said, *"Mamacita,* today is Thanksgiving Day and we are eating together, we all share food. Let's go eat." As I put my hand out for her, we walked back to her chair and sat her down.

To my relief, *mamacita* resumed eating her meal. To my surprise, five minutes later, she got up from her chair again and repeated this scene. I, too, got up rapidly and went to her as I did earlier. I noted this time, she was somewhat reluctant to sit down and I quickly prayed for guidance. As I grabbed her arm, she looked around with a dazed look as if she was lost. I also noted the number of people in the room seemed to irritate her and she did not seem to recognize they were her *familia*. In retrospect, I can now say, I did not realize that due to her illness, she was not able to cope with any large crowd, even though it was small and even though it was her *familia*. Please note, this incident was the **first** time she had acted this way around *la familia*. Strange to say, but this was reality and it hit us right in our faces! I was embarrassed and sad for her and us that Alzheimer's had progressed this far. Later that night, I concluded we would not be able to celebrate any happy occasions like Thanksgiving Day with my mother anymore. I felt real sad. As one can imagine, there went our appetite! We did not talk about it anymore, we were all frozen in our seats and I decided to take *mi mamacita* to her home immediately. It was a most interesting drive; I never mentioned the incident nor did she. It did not matter though she had already forgotten about it!

Personal Suggestions

Please know your loved one's limitations; Alzheimer's has different stages; family must be aware and prepared for changes in their loved ones' mental status. Bringing *mamacita* to one's home may not be the best idea even though one desires to do so. Be prepared! Good luck!

Thanksgiving Day #2
(*Otro Día de dar Gracias*)

This one occurred a year later. Of course, I remembered what had happened the year before, give me a break! That is why this one is very different. Obviously as a daughter, I still wanted my *familia* to enjoy our *mamacita*. After all, I am a stubborn daughter. I love *familia*, holidays and I was determined to have turkey with them. I decided, this time, *mi familia* was going to have the party at our mamacita's house. Along with that, of course, better planning had to be done because all the food had to be taken to her house. I informed the family as I always did. San Antonio, here we go again! My younger sister from Houston donated the turkey and Tony and I donated the rest of the goodies. I was excited because we would continue to celebrate Thanksgiving Day with my mother as family should.

Party Day Arrived (*Llego el Día de Party*)

At about 5 P.M. in the afternoon, my husband and I, my family, my brother and his family arrived at my mother's house for dinner. Our *mamacita* greeted us warmly at her house and said "*¿Que estan haciendo ustedes aquí?*" (what are we doing here?) I told her it was Thanksgiving Day and we were having dinner at her house. She smiled and excitedly said, "That is nice." We visited with *mi mamacita* patiently for over an hour. After an hour or so later, we asked ourselves, where is the turkey? A little while later, a white Surburban is outside the door. Everyone knows, including our *mamacita*, that it is Liza with her daughters. We all went out to the car to greet her and to help carry the turkey and the rest of the "goodies." To our surprise, Liza jumped out and brought out a large ice chest on wheels, boxes, pots and pans. I looked into the Suburban to look for the turkey to take inside the house and could not find it. Hmmm . . . I wondered to myself, where is the turkey? For a moment, I thought that Liza was playing games with us and most especially with our *mamacita*. I asked Liza, where is the turkey and she said, "The turkey is in the ice chest." The ice chest, I exclaimed! How could a turkey fit in the ice chest, I wondered. I stood there puzzled and asked her again, "Where is the turkey?" She ignored me and continued to unpack and I have to say, she probably did not hear me or she was throwing me for crazy or playing games with us, because she did not respond. *Mamacita* and I just laughed and continued looking frantically but we still could not find it. Okay, I said to myself, I do not understand, I just have to ask Liza again. *Mi mamacita* and I both shouted, "*Liza, where is the turkey?*" Liza smiled, laughed and said, "The turkey is in the ice chest in the baggies!" Baggies, I exclaimed! What, no way, I cannot believe that, show me the turkey Liza, I said! I could not understand how a 20 lb. Turkey could be in a baggie? I thought, what has this world turned into?

After a few minutes of intense laughter by all of *mi familia*, my sister explained she had sliced and separated portions of the turkey for her other family in Houston. We laughed so much to the extent tears flowed from our eyes. Leave a situation like this to Liza, I thought. She was the funny one of the family, of course, and she proved it again! None of us had ever seen a turkey in a baggie. I have to add, it was not the same, seeing a turkey in a baggie compared to seeing it complete. Oh, well!

I think that the whole family will always remember

this particular Thanksgiving Day because it was a First in our books! Yea, we were all glad that the turkey did taste good after all. Oh well! This particular Thanksgiving Day story has been shared with a lot of family for many years. It was a fun dinner/party and *mi mamacita* enjoyed the closeness of her *familia* at her house. She did not lose her temper, which was wonderful. We were blessed! *Gracias a Dios* (Thanks be to God).

The moral of the story is to enjoy the holidays with your *mamacita* or your loved one while she/he can still enjoy and understand what is going on, kind of/sort of!

Personal Summary Suggestions

Educate and prepare yourself in advance. You must know your loved one. Try to predict how she will react in family gatherings but at the same time, you must be patient and flexible for changes. Good luck!

Story #3 of Thanksgiving Day

After moving her to the condo, Thanksgiving was drastically different. We had to adjust again and again. I truly had to evaluate *mamacita's* mood before I decided how we were to celebrate this special day. Sometimes, I took her to my brother's house and fed her immediately and then took her and the sitter back to the condo immediately after the meal. This way, she too had Thanksgiving with *mi familia*. After she returned back to the condo, *mi familia* continued the dinner and everyone was happy. That is our modern day Thanksgiving Day celebration. This seems to work so far and we will enjoy this as long as we can. I am aware that *mamacita*'s mental capacity will deteriorate so I am going to celebrate with *mi mamacita* as long as I can. There were other Thanksgiving days whereby I went to the condo and took her and the sitter a plate full of turkey and trimmings. Whatever works, that is my motto!

Merry Christmas and a Happy New Year!
(¡*Feliz Navidad y Prospero Año Nuevo!*)

Happy Holidays everybody!!! It may not be the holiday season when one reads this book, but that is okay. We are welcome to dream and think about all the wonderful holidays in our past, our present and our future (*con familia y amigos*) with families and friends. We can think about the snows we have had or as far as that goes, down in San Antonio, Texas, the snows we rarely had. We can also think about those presents we have received and the presents we have not received, and the presents that we may have recycled. We can think about the children and their smiles when they have seen their presents and the beautiful, green decorated Christmas tree and all the decorations. Oh, how pretty! Oh, yea, we can dream . . . that is okay. Oh well, we can enjoy the many blessings we all have been given with health, family and friends.

First of all, I would like to thank my dear God for all the years he has given me with *mi mamacita*. Also, for all our (*familia y amigos*) families and friends. I am trying to express to everyone, since my mother's Alzheimer's has progressed, all of the joyous holidays will never be the same. But, we must not get depressed but work with the situation because we are *familia*. I will admit though, it

205

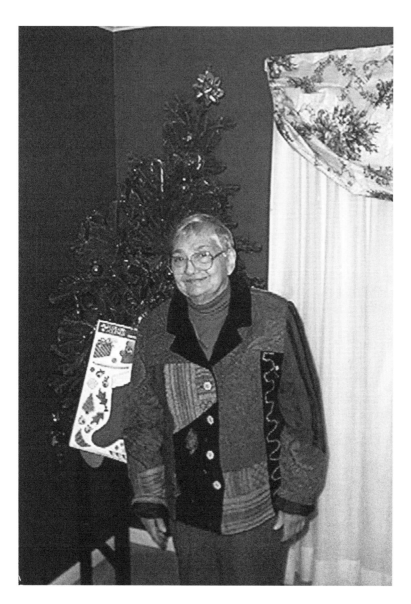

Mi Mamacita

206

has been extremely difficult for *mi familia* to enjoy the true meaning of the holidays.

I would like to pay a special holiday tribute to *mi mamacita* and all caregivers, families and loved ones with Alzheimer's, with a memory flashback of my past holidays. Maybe you too can do this. Now, close your eyes and remember Christmas as a child. Wow, how beautiful, I hope!

As a child and coming from a large family, oh yea, we had wonderful Christmases every year. My parents decorated the outside of the house with lights and of course the Christmas tree too. Yearly, we went out to buy a live tree from the grocery store. *Mi mamacita* decorated and filled it with presents for us children. I remember Christmas very well because it was so much fun. It was so beautiful! The house, the tree, the presents, the food and midnight Mass of course. Yes, *mi mamacita* cooked a delicious meal and we gathered to eat dinner like *familia*. Dinner consisted of ham and turkey and a lot of other "goodies." After dinner, we opened the presents.

As we grew up and married, our dinner parties kept getting bigger and bigger due to the large number of children and grandchildren around. Our happy times continued until *mamacita* got sick with her Alzheimer's. Oh yes, we have been blessed with many wonderful holidays including Christmas. *Gracias a Dios* (Thanks be to God).

I am sad to say those happy days are gone forever. She cannot tolerate crowds nor noise and has forgotten her manners. Now, please forgive me for what I am going to tell you about *mi mamacita* and her Alzheimer's, but I must. I want everyone to understand that Alzheimer's robs our loved one from *familia*.But please remember, they need love because they are *familia* too. In a way, it kind of sounds like a disclaimer. Some of this stuff is not

207

proper for one's ears, but here comes a large dose of reality.

Mi mamacita expresses signs of aggression by her outbursts of voice and behavior. She shouts and cusses occasionally. Her paranoia toward people, even to *familia,* has progressed quite a bit. She stares at people and checks and rechecks doors. She accuses people of eating and stealing her food. She makes people and *familia* uncomfortable by this behavior. Our *mamacita* has drastically changed forever and the holidays will never be the same. Currently, we have tried to continue to celebrate the holidays *con mi mamacita*, of course with modifications. *Mi mamacita* now spends Christmas with her sitter and a limited number of *familia*. We visit and try to continue to celebrate this and all special holidays with *mamacita* the best that we can.

My goal for *mi mamacita* is to continue to share the holidays with her as long as I can. I will try to accomplish this to the extent as much as possible for whatever life she has left. I will try to make them fun, safe and comfortable because she is *mi mamacita*.

Thank you, God, for *mi mamacita*.

19

My Return to Washington

After living with *mi mamacita* twenty-four hours a day, seven days a week for one whole month, I concluded the best way I could help her was to be the coordinator of her care. I quickly learned she did not need me to sit with her twenty-four hours a day; she needed me differently. She needed me to be alert, rested and able to make decisions at a drop of a dime and without any hesitation and pronto. Therefore, I planned my move back to the Washington, D.C. area almost as soon as I arrived like I was taught back in Nursing School, which was to start to plan early for proper facilitation. But, I always kept the final goal in mind; to ensure *mi mamacita* remained comfortable, safe and happy in San Antonio, Texas.

As a daughter, her guardian and her nurse, I needed to continue to coordinate all of her care on a short-and-long-distance basis. I had no doubt with my decision. I concluded that a caregiver does not have to live with a loved one with Alzheimer's 24/7 to accomplish this goal. It is just different. One is always responsible! The following are factors coordinated in planning my move back to Washington, D.C.: Day care, doctor and dentist visits along with sitter arrangements for 24/7 coverage and my brother to continue his weekly visit. The *magic* words in providing care are coordinate, flexibility, patience, love, faith, determination and *familia*. That is all! Last but not least, I had to ensure I had enough money to pay for these sitters by speaking with family about the sale of her home. I accomplished this through communication of e-mail as enclosed:

Sample of E-mail to Family
Subject: Mother's Carelink

Dear family! Hello to all and hope that all are doing fine. This is an update on mother! GREAT NEWS! Jesse and Josie, our cousins from California, have recently bought Mother's house. They are very excited since Jesse has fond memories of being born there. The money will continue to provide for mother's care for sitters (agency) for 24/7 which is what she needs. As a result, I am moving back to Virginia (D.C. area) to continue to live with my husband and go back to my nursing career since I have accomplished my goal here of ensuring that MOM is safe, comfortable, happy and has 24/7 coverage to ensure this! I would like to thank the family members who helped me accomplish this goal (through money, calls and cards) and may God bless you all! I will continue to pay for the condo and its dues. I will continue to call her twice daily and visit quarterly or more often as necessary. Mom will pay for the sitters, groceries, utility bills and my airline/visits to ensure of her safety. Mom will continue to go to day care. She smiles more and even says thank-you; acknowledges that she is happy; loves the small day trips including to the fast food restaurants that the day care, Liza, Tony, sitters and myself have taken her to. She is stable physically but is deteriorating slowly mentally. She recognizes the regular family members, sometimes! She is saying the wrong words and phrases for things, i.e. The water is not hot when she really means turn off the faucet. She wants to wash her face with mouthwash; she can't bathe nor dress herself, cook, etc. (One really needs to spend time with her to really understand what she means and how to care for a loved one with Alzheimer's.) That is why she needs 24/7 sitters! She is not SAFE to herself! I am blessed and very happy that I had the opportunity to have enjoyed our MOM and provide a safe, happy and comfortable home for her even though her mind is deteriorating. I thank GOD for all those family members that have helped MOM and will continue to help MOM to care for her at the condo! I would like to ask the other family members to PLEASE RECONSIDER to help MOM because she will lose all of her mind, her funny smiles, laughter and herself in the coming days, months, and we do not know how much time she will bless us with her presence here on Earth! THANKS AGAIN to the family members that are helping MOM and may GOD bless you! Please continue to send money, or save it until next summer WHEN THE MONEY RUNS OUT!! Please continue to call her, send greeting cards, pray and remember her. Please do not send her money, send me the money because she will lose it.

My best to all! Love, Terry

That same night, after I sent the above e-mail, I packed my luggage. The next morning, bright and early, I told *mi mamacita* I was going back to work in Washington and she said, "That is nice." After breakfast Clara, the sitter, *mi mamacita* and I got into the car, and I drove to the airport. Mother just smiled and did not say a word. No one said a word. When we arrived at the airport, I got out, kissed her and told her I had to go to work. She asked me,

"¿*Vas a regresar?*" (are you coming back?) I said, "Yes" and she looked content with my response. I was happy with a peacefulness in my heart, I left her with a piece of mind that she was safe, comfortable and happy, as I felt. I felt that I had completed my goal and I would continue to care for *mi mamacita* As I walked into the airport, I did not look back. As of this date, I continue to accomplish my responsibility of being a daughter and a nurse. I continue to coordinate all of her care. *Gracias a Dios* (Thanks be to God). ¡*Que Dios los bendigá a todos los queridos con Alzheimer's y todos que los cudan*! (May God bless all those loved ones with Alzheimer's and the caregivers too!)

In summary, I returned to the Washington, D.C. area to accomplish both responsibilities of *mi mamacita* and my husband. I prayed for guidance and assistance in making this decision. I concluded that I could take care of *mi mamacita* on a long distance basis. Living with *mi mamacita* gave me a better appreciation and inspiration of her and of all the other loved Alzheimer's patients in the world. It has further opened my eyes and I continue to enjoy her as long as my God lends her to *mi familia*. I learned that everyday I lived with *mi mamacita* was different and I *am* a very lucky and blessed daughter to have been given this "gift." Life is a very precious gift, just like taking care of one's *mamacita* is a very special gift. If you are given this "gift," do the best that you can with it. If you're not given this gift, then support your *familia*; they need your moral as well as financial support because this is what *familia* is all about. Do it for *amor, fé y familia* (love, faith and family).

I would like to share with you my daily phone log. On the next few pages are Samples: **I must pre-alert everyone that I love to make my *mamacita* laugh and therefore I started my conversations with comedy.**

MORNINGS: (Here Is a Sample of Our Three Phone Calls)

(1)

ME: "Good morning, Ma'am, is this Taco Hut? Are you open?"

MOM: "Hello ma'am, yes, this is Taco Hut, it is open, what is it that you want?"

ME: "I would like 500 tacos."

MOM: . . . chuckle . . . "500 tacos, oh no, that is too many tacos."

ME: "Oh ma'am, you are the Queen, you can make 500 tacos, I know that you can. After all, you are my *mamacita* and you cook the best tacos."

MOM: chuckle . . . "I am your *mamacita,* that is nice."

ME: We both chuckle . . . "Hello *Mamacita,* how are you?"

MOM: "Oh, I don't feel good, I have a headache." (NOTE: She always has a headache.)

ME: "I am so sorry, maybe you need to lie down and rest a little."

MOM: "Okay, I will lie down. Will that take my headache away?"

ME: "Yes, Mother, your headache will go away if you rest. Go ahead and lie down. I will call you later when you feel better."

MOM: "Thank you for calling."

(2)

ME: "Good morning, ma'am, is this Taco Hut? Are you open this beautiful morning?"

MOM: "Good morning, ma'am, let me find out if we are open. Are we open? Yes, we are open. What is it that you want?"

ME: "I want 500 tacos."

MOM: chuckle . . . "Who is this? What do you want?"

ME: "It is your favorite daughter, Terry, and I want you, *Mamacita.*"

MOM: chuckle . . . "Oh, you silly girl. So you are my daughter?"

ME: "Yes, I am silly and yes, I am your daughter."

MOM: "If you are my daughter why are you not here?"

ME: "I live in Washington, mom, with my husband, Juan."

MOM: "You live in Washington with your husband, I didn't know that."

ME: "Yes, I live in Washington with my husband. How are you?"

MOM: "I feel okay today."

ME: "Wonderful, I am happy that you feel good today."

MOM: "You feel wonderful, that is nice, I feel wonderful too."

ME: "Yes, that is nice. How is the weather?"

MOM: "The weather is raining." (NOTE: it is not raining.)

ME: "What are do doing, mother?"

MOM: "I am relaxing."

ME: "That is nice, I am glad that you are relaxing."

MOM: "Yes, I am relaxing."

214

ME: "Mom, have you had a bath yet? You know I like to smell you because you smell nice after a bath."

MOM: "You like to smell me? That is nice. Yes, I already took a bath."

ME: Yes, Mom, that is nice. I have to go to work. Be a good girl and have a nice day."

MOM: "You too, be a good girl."

ME: "I will call you tonight."

MOM: "Okay, good-bye, don't forget to call."

ME: "Nope, I will not forget to call, good-bye."

(3)

ME: "Good morning, ma'am, is this Taco Hut? Are you open?"

MOM: "Hello ma'am, yes, this is Taco Hut and it is open, what is it that you want?"

ME: "I would like 500 tacos."

MOM: . . . chuckle . . . "500 tacos, oh no, that is too many tacos."

ME: "Oh, Mom, I am just joking, I just like to hear you laugh. You sound so nice when you laugh."

MOM: "I sound happy when I laugh?"

ME: "Yes, Mom, you sound happy. Are you happy, Mom?"

MOM: "Yes, I am happy."

ME: Wonderful, I want you to be happy"

MOM: "Yes, I am happy."

ME: "What are you doing, *mamacita?*"

MOM: "I am cleaning the house." (NOTE: She cannot clean the house.)

ME: "Great, I am glad that you are cleaning the

house. My house needs cleaning and I am happy that you are helping me clean the house."

MOM: "Yes, I am happy that you are happy to clean the house."

ME: "Thank you for cleaning the house, *mamacita*."

MOM: "You are welcome. I gotta go now, good-bye."

ME: "You gotta go, where are you going?"

MOM: "I gotta go, good-bye. I gotta go and take care of the children."

ME: "Okay, Mom, say hello to the children for me. Take care of yourself."

EVENINGS: (More Phone Calls)

(1)

ME: "Hello, is this Pizza Hut? Is it still open?"

MOM: "Hello, yes, this is Pizza Hut. Yes, we are still open. We are almost ready to close, what is it that you want?"

ME: "Ma'am, I would like 500 pizzas."

MOM: "500 pizzas! Oh no, that is too many pizzas."

ME: "But ma'am, can you make me five pizzas instead?"

MOM: "Yes . . . but we have no pizzas." Chuckle. . . .

ME: (We both laugh). " *Mamacita,* how are you tonight?"

MOM: "I am fine, I am glad that you called. Where are you? Why are you not here where I can see you? I want to go home."

ME: "*Mamacita,* I am in Washington, D.C. right now, I cannot come right now."

MOM: "I didn't know that. When are you coming?"

ME: "I will come down in one month to visit you."

MOM: "That is nice that you are coming down to see me. Then can you take me home?"

ME: "Yes, then I will take you home." (NOTE: Due to Alzheimer's, she always wants to go home for the comfort as a child.)

MOM: "That is good, I will wait for you."

ME: "How was your day today? Did you go anywhere today?" (NOTE: she goes to day care three days a week.)

MOM: "No, I did not go anywhere today, I stayed home all day. I am upset with your dad because he has not called. You know your dad, he can be stubborn." (NOTE: My dad has been deceased for over four years now.)

ME: "Mom, don't worry about Dad, I will check on him. I will take care of that. I don't want you to worry. That is my job to worry for you. Okay, Mother?"

MOM: "Okay, *mejita* (daughter), I will not worry."

ME: "What are you doing, Mother?"

MOM: "I am watching TV."

ME: "Are you watching *novellas*?" (soap operas in Spanish).

MOM: "No, I am watching something. I don't remember what it is. But they are making a lot of noise."

ME: "Okay, Mother, you have a good night. Don't forget to say your prayers."

MOM: "I won't. You don't forget to say yours too. Thank you for calling."

ME: "Good night, Mother."

MOM: "Good night."

(2)

ME: "Hello, is this Pizza Hut? Is it still open?"
MOM: "Hello, yes, this is Pizza Hut. Let me find out
if we are still open. Yes, we are still open. We are
almost ready to close, what is it that you want?
You are lucky that we are still open."
ME: "Ma'am, I would like 500 pizzas."
MOM: "500 pizzas! Oh no, pizzas we do not have."
ME: "Hello, Mother, how are you this afternoon?"
MOM: "I want to go home. I am scared here. I am
afraid that someone is coming by and kill me. I
do not understand what is going on. Everyone is
strange. There is no one here, I am by myself."
ME: "Mother, I understand that things are strange,
but it is your mind. It is playing games. Do you
trust me? You must trust me. I love you and I
will take care of you. The lady next to you is my
friend. She is helping me to take care of you. You
will NEVER be alone. NO one will ever hurt you.
You must pray and have faith. You must believe
me."
MOM: "Yes, I trust you. Yes, I have faith. Yes, I will
pray. Are you sure that no one will hurt me?"
ME: "Yes, MOM, I am sure that no one will hurt you
and you must trust me. The house has an alarm
and the police check the neighborhoods frequently. You must trust me."
MOM: "Yes, I trust you."
ME: "How is the weather? Is the sun still out?"
MOM: "No, it is dark outside and I am sleepy."
ME: "I guess it is night-time and time for bed. Well,
goodnight and don't forget to say your prayers."
MOM: "Good night."

(3)

ME: "Hello, ma'am, is this Pizza Hut? Are you still open?"

MOM: chuckle . . . "Yes, this is Pizza Hut and we are closed. You need to call earlier."

ME: "Oh, ma'am, I am so very, very hungry, what do you suggest that I do?"

MOM: "Eat your *pata* (foot)."

ME: "Oh, you silly mother. . . . How are you tonight?"

MOM: "I'm okay tonight."

ME: "I'm so happy that you are fine tonight."

MOM: "You are happy?"

ME: "Yes, I am happy. I want you to be happy. Are you happy?"

MOM: "Yes, I am happy."

ME: "Good, now that we are both happy, what are you doing?"

MOM: "I am just laying down on my bed and reading a book." (NOTE: she does not like to read anymore.)

ME: "Good, reading is good for the brain, it makes you smarter."

MOM: "I didn't know that."

ME: "How was your day today?"

MOM: "I had a nice day."

ME: "Good, well, I better go now, you be a good girl, say your prayers and go to sleep."

MOM: "I will, you do too. Will you call me tomorrow?"

ME: "Yes, I will call you every day."

MOM: "Good, I want you to call me. Good night."

(4)

ME: "Hello *mamacita,* are you my sweet mama?"

MOM: "Hello, yes, I am your sweet mama" Chuckle
. . . "What is it that you want?"

ME: "I just want to hear your pretty voice and make
you laugh."

MOM: "You say I have a pretty voice, that is nice."

ME: "How are you, pretty mama?"

MOM: "I don't feel good, a FISH bit me today on my
arm."

ME: "A FISH bit you? WOW!! You better go lie down
and rest so the pain can go away."

MOM: "Are you sure I will feel better?"

ME: "Yes, I am sure you will feel better."

MOM: "Okay, good night."

ME: "Good night *mamacita,* be a good girl. I will call
you tomorrow."

I am very sad to say, this last sample definitely
shows the reader *mamacita*'s deteriorating mental
changes:

ME: Hello, hello, *mamacita*, how are you? It is I,
Terry, your daughter.

MOM: No response. (I am told by the sitter that *mi
mamacita* is eating the telephone. (This is so
sad!)

Boy, let me tell you, this FISH STORY, sure puts to
competition all those FISH stories that we all hear. Oh
dear Lord, give me guidance *y paciencia* (and patience)!

220

Routine Life of *Mi Mamacita*

Mamacita continued to go to Day Care three times a week for about three years, then she stopped walking. Occasionally, she showed periods of aggression with her sitters by her cuss words XXXXX but these symptoms have not progressed Amen!

Currently, I am at peace. I know I am doing the best I can on a long distance basis. I know this chapter of my life with *mi mamacita* continues on a daily basis. I know I need to go back home to care for her when her condition deteriorates, but until then, I am spiritually at peace and I will be there in a flash physically with the help of the airlines and a speeding phone call. We, her *familia,* are definitely blessed she is presently cruising to the best of her ability. *Gracias a Dios* (Thanks be to God).

For about a year, life seemed to have cruised by without any major obstacle with *mi mamacita* in San Antonio, Texas with sitters and I in the East Coast until her money ran out. Money run out, one might wonder, how can that be? Well, it definitely does cost money to pay to live, especially private pay sitters. Then I thought, it was time for plan B, whatever that was! It was called reality check! After consultation with my husband, my siblings, Lisa and Tony, I asked the other family members for their financial support to continue to provide quality care for our *mamacita.*

Here is a copy of the family e-mail.

HAPPY MOTHER'S DAY!!! Dear Brothers, Sisters and Mother's Grandchildren. This is an update on Mother's care. As of July 1, 2003, all of MOM's and DAD's funds will be used up to pay the agency that provides 24/7 care for MOM. This means that MOM is in a FINANCIAL CRISIS!!! Mom's monthly annuity is $590 and goes to pay her food, medicines and utilities. Mom's care giver agency charges an average of $3,300 per month which is $110/day. Once all the funds are depleted, (7/1/03), Lisa, Tony, Debbie, Sylvia and I have agreed to contribute funds to help pay on a monthly basis to continue to provide quality care for MOM. This is obviously a sacrifice and a burden on all of us. I respectfully hope and pray that you find it in your heart and mind to help out MOM. MOM would gladly appreciate any amount, even $25, $50, $100 or more on a monthly basis. Please respond ASAP so MOM can continue to receive quality care. Thank you! May God bless you!

BILLS: (monthly)		INCOME: (As of 7/1/03-Monthly)	
Medicines	$250	Dad/Mom's Annuity:	$590
Agency Sitters	$3,330	Debbie	$100
Food	$200	Lisa	$500
Utilities	$150	Sylvia	$400
TOTAL:	$3,900	Tony	$500
		Terry	$500
		TOTAL:	2,590

NEED: $1,310 MORE to continue to provide for MOM's care

Please note that this letter will be mailed to all family members in addition to e-mail. Please also, if you know that someone does not have an e-mail address, please feel free to advertise to them so that MOM's care can be continued.

Take care and hello to everyone!! THANK YOU! Love, Terry

I received several financial challenges from some family members and I thank those for their financial assistance and their love and devotion. May God bless them. *Gracias a Dios.* (Thanks to God.)

20

Epilogue

Hey everybody, update time! My, my, how time has flown by! Presently I live in the Washington, D.C. area and have continued my responsibilities as a long-distance caregiver. It continues to be challenging, loving, and invigorating. I call *mi mamacita* daily even though the conversation does not make sense. I am most sure I can write many, many more stories of *mi mamacita* until my beloved *Dios* (God) takes her to Heaven. Caring for *mi mamacita* has been interesting and most "rewarding" to be quite honest. I truly believe this has been my "calling." I also believe *mi mamacita* is alive by the grace of our dear Lord. I really don't know how she "trucks along" but only God knows, and I have learned not to question "**Him**" anymore. *Mi mamacita* continues to amaze me every single day with the beauty of her smile and laughter, even though her mind is in another world. Her behavior has changed drastically; she is now a "chatterbox," is incontinent, and has difficulty walking. She is a total care person. Many times, I feel sad for her and of her deteriorating mental condition because she is not aware of it. At the same time I feel so very sad this has happened to *mi mamacita* because she is *mi mamacita*! Caring for *mi mamacita* has not been an easy task, but I can handle it, thanks to God. I strongly believe God does not give us something one cannot handle. Of course, it has been difficult and challenging. Yes, of course, sometimes, when I feel sad, I pray and ask God for strength and guidance to help me cope and accept this challenge. I would like to thank all of *mi mamacita*'s family who gave their love and finances out of the kindness of their hearts and who continue caring for our *mamacita!*

I will conclude this story with the following: "The purpose of life, after all, is to live it, to taste experience to the utmost, to reach out eagerly and without fear for newer and richer experience." Eleanor Roosevelt.[11]

Appendix
Favorite Mexican Sayings
(*Dichos/Chistos*)

Dichos to my Hispanic/Latino people are like jokes or sayings. These make us smile and laugh as they are part of my everyday culture. I would love to share some *dichos* that I grew up with:

- When your hand itches, it means you will get some money soon,
- When you have a ringworm, it means you are a thief,
- When you stutter, go see if the birds are flying and go stand outside,
- *Cuando tengas un susto, ponga un huevo abajo de la cama* (When you are scared, put an egg under your bed),
- *Cuando tienes un dolor del estomado, ponga aceste y massagelo* (when you have a stomach ache, put some lard and massage it in),
- *Todo en la vida se puede recuperar, pero el tiempo nunca se recuperar* (You can recover everything in life but time),
- *La familia primero* (the family comes first),
- *Hay que tener respecto* (you must be respectful),
- *Hay que aguanar* (you must tolerate, accept),

- *Hay espiritus malos* (there are bad things or evils),
- *Cuidate* (be careful),
- *Respecto* (respect).

More *Dichos*

Dios no nos dar algo que no podemos hacer, estamos calgardo Nuestra Cruz. (God does not give us something that we cannot handle, we are carrying our cross). (Unknown author),

Dalé gas (Give it gas) (Unknown author),

Querer es poder (When there's a will there is a way),[2]

Al buen entendedor, Pocas Palabras (To those apt to understand, few words),[2]

Cuando joven, de ilusiones: cuando Viejo de recuerdos (While young, one dreams; when old, all memories).[2]

I would hope some of you can remember other *dichos* too! Please smile and enjoy!

Bibliography

This list features only the books that I have used as a reference. There are MANY, MANY wonderful reference books that are helpful, supportive and educational for the person who wants to learn about Alzheimer's and its proper care:

1. Alzheimer's Association, Free Brochures in English/Spanish on Alzheimer's; care for the patient and for the Caregiver. (Can be obtained from the national or local chapters) 1-800-272-3900. www.aiz.org
2. Sellers, Jeff M. *Folk Wisdom of Mexico, Proverbios y dichos Mexicanos,* Chronicle Books.
3. Nava, Yolanda. *It's All in the Frijoles,* A Fireside Book, Simon & Schuster.
4. Grace Place Day Care, Multiple hand-outs and support group, San Antonio, Texas.
5. National Family Caregivers Association, Brochure: *"10 Tips on Family Caregivers,"* and other Caregiver information. 1-800-896-3650/www.thefamilycaregiver.org
6. Lewis, Sharon, RN, PhD, FAAN, *"Stress-Busting Program for Caregivers,"* University of Texas Health Science Center, San Antonio, Texas.
7. Delgado, Jane, Ph.D., M.S., *Salud,* Rayo, Harper Collins.
8. Gray-Davidson, Grena, *The Alzheimer's Sourcebook for Caregivers,* Lowell House.
9. *A Time for Alzheimer's,* Florence Baurys, RN, Elmerald Ink Pubishers.
10. *The 36-Hour Day,* Nancy L. Mace, MA and Peter V.

Rabbins, MD, MPH, A Johns Hopkins Press Health Book. (printed in English and Spanish).
11. *Chicken Soup for the Golden Soul,* Jack Canfield, Mark Victor Hansen, Paul J. Meyer, Barbara Russell Chesser and Amy Seeger. Health Communications, Inc.
12. *Failure Free Activities for the Alzheimer's Patient,* Sheridan Carmel, Cottage Books.
13. *Coping with Caring, Daily Reflections for the Alzheimer's Caregiver,* Lyn Roche, Elder Books.
14. Vicente Fernandez—CD's.

About the Author

Mary Theresa Schultz Vasquez RN (Terry) was born and raised in San Antonio, Texas and currently resides in the Washington, D.C. area. She is the sixth child of nine children, comes from a typical large, Hispanic/Latina family of her day. Since her childhood, she was nicknamed Terry and has used it ever since. Upon marriage, she took her husband's last name of Vasquez, which is in the Hispanic/Latina tradition and has proudly used it for over thirty-five years.

Ms. Vasquez has been a Registered Nurse for over thirty-five years and has worked in almost all facets of nursing including the hospital setting in Texas, California, New York, and Virginia. She also worked as the Events Liaison for the Hispanic Heritage Foundation, a non-profit organization in Washington, D.C. and with Inova Health Systems in Northern Virginia as a Home Health Nurse. She currently works as an Immunization Nurse with Health Source Inova Health Systems in Northern Virginia.

Ms. Vasquez graduated from San Antonio College in San Antonio, Texas with an Associates Degree in Nursing. She is a member of the American Nurses Association, the Virginia Nurses Association, the National Association of Hispanic Nurses, the National Alzheimer's Association as well as other chapters.

She is also a member of the National Family Caregivers Association and a State Representative for Virginia. In 2003, she served on a Task Force for the "End of Life Issues," symposium in San Antonio, Texas. Ms. Vasquez is also a member of Las Comadres para las Americas and MANA, a national Latina organization.

Acknowledgments include:

- Certificate of Recognition for ten years of dedicated service, Inova Health System, Fairfax, Virginia.
- Employee of the Month, 1990, St. Luke's Lutheran Hospital, San Antonio, Texas.
- Honorable mention-Honor Roll, October 1980, *The Teaching Post*, (Newsletter of the Nursing Service Patient Education Committee), Houston Veterans Administration Medical Center, Houston, Texas.

Ms. Vasquez is a Registered Nurse because her father wanted her to be one. During the writing of this book, Ms. Vasquez resided in San Antonio, Texas on a full-time basis. Ms. Vasquez cared for her mother due to a "calling."